TRUE LYME

Understanding, Treating, and Thriving with
Lyme Disease: A Comprehensive Guide

JOHN FROUDE MD FRCP

*"Do not allow thirst for profit, ambition for renown and admiration, to
interfere with my profession for these are enemies of truth"*
Maimonides, physician.

AuthorHouse™ UK
1663 Liberty Drive
Bloomington, IN 47403 USA
www.authorhouse.co.uk
UK TFN: 0800 0148641 (Toll Free inside the UK)
UK Local: 02036 956322 (+44 20 3695 6322 from outside the UK)

This book is printed on acid-free paper.

ISBN: 979-8-8230-8355-3 (sc)
ISBN: 979-8-8230-8357-7 (hc)
ISBN: 979-8-8230-8356-0 (e)

Library of Congress Control Number: 2023912958

Print information available on the last page.

Published by AuthorHouse 11/08/2023

authorHOUSE®

Dedicated to Elaine Taylor and Marshall Berland.

Table of Contents

NINE TRUTHS ABOUT LYME

1. THE TYPICAL RASH IS NOT A BULL'S EYE

2. IT WAS FIRST DESCRIBED IN SWEDEN IN 1912, NOT LYME, CONNECTICUT IN 1975

3. THE LYME ANTIBODY TEST IS NEGATIVE FOR THE FIRST TWO TO EIGHT WEEKS AFTER INFECTION

4. NO DIAGNOSIS OF DEMENTIA IS ACCEPTABLE UNTIL LYME HAS BEEN EXCLUDED

5. AS LYME IS POTENTIALLY CURABLE IT SHOULD ALWAYS BE CONSIDERED IN THE DIFFERENTIAL DIAGNOSIS

6. EARLY DIAGNOSIS IS ESSENTIAL

7. CO-INFECTIONS MUST BE LOOKED FOR AND TREATED

8. IT HAS OCCURED IN ALL FIFTY OF THE UNITED STATES

9. IF IN DOUBT, TREAT

And as a bonus, ITS NAME IS LYME DISEASE NOT *LYME'S* DISEASE
It is named after a place not a person.

PROLOGUE

Ötzi the Iceman's torso was found sticking out of a glacier high on a mountainside in the Austrian Tyrol near the Italian border. His whole body had been mummified by nature. A couple of German hikers found him in 1991. His corpse had lain there for 5,300 years since he had died in his 40s.

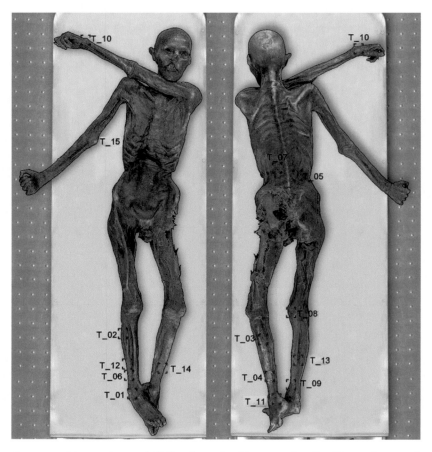

Courtesy: Marco Samadelli/Institute for Mummy Studies/Eurac Research

Much would be learned from his body and his possessions. He had over a hundred tattoos on him, simple designs placed mostly over joints. In his stomach was food from a recent meal that included venison. He had a copper axe and a bow, a deerskin quiver containing flint pointed arrows. It was a blow to the head of unknowable cause that killed him.

His human DNA had features detectable in a group of modern-day Austrians who lived in the valley below. It also showed that he had genes for lactose intolerance and high cholesterol.
Bacterial DNA was also found in the mix. It came from the genus known as *Spirochetae*. It was identified as *Borrelia burgdorferi* the bacteria that causes a disease well recognized on the Eastern seaboard of the United States in the twenty first Century.

Ötzi was the first human known to have Lyme disease.

Part One
THE ILLNESS

Chapter One
ACUTE LYME
THE THREAT IN THE YARD

When an infected deer tick bites you it injects *Borrelia burgdorferi* (*Bb*), a bacteria, into your skin which makes its way to your bloodstream. Your immune system is triggered, and an acute inflammatory response follows to try and kick it out.

Lyme does *not* cause shaking chills and very high fevers. Throughout its course it is laid back, it is *subacute*. Other bacteria, such as *Anaplasmosis*, transmitted by the same tick that transmits *Bb*, are more aggressive.

Yet you are undoubtedly ill with weakness, malaise, poor appetite, aches and pains in your muscles and joints to go with your low-grade fever. It's like the flu. You may take to your bed.

It's been 3 to 30 days since the tick bit you and wherever it did you may notice a red spot, 5-20 cm in diameter. It can be anywhere on your body but areas where you might not notice a tick such as the hairline or behind your knee or in your armpit or on your back are more common. The tick would need to be attached to you for at least 24 hours before it injects *Bb* into you and if it were in a more obvious place such as on your forearm you might pull or rub it off.

The medical term for the big red spot is Erythema Chronicum Migrans (ECM). This unwieldy phrase is taken from the earliest description of the disease in Europe. Erythema means red. Chronicum is Latin for chronic. It fades over three weeks. Migrans might make you think it migrates about the body but it doesn't, it spreads out from the spot where the tick bit you. Still, to call it an ECM is a useful shorthand. Very often the C is dropped, and the spot is called an EM.

In case you find the same term used to describe certain lesions of the tongue those have nothing to do with Lyme.

In popular speech it is called the "bullseye" or "typical bullseye rash".

These are some examples of the typical rash of Lyme and as you can see, it is NOT a bullseye.

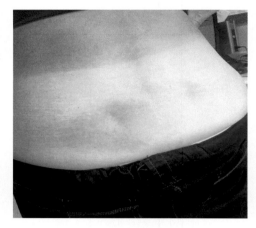

This is the typical rash of Lyme.

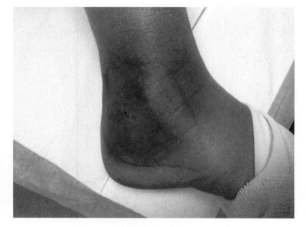

Note how red and angry it looks, but it does not hurt. Sometimes patients complain of itchiness or mild pain.

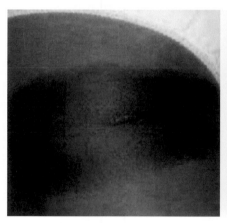

This patient was not even aware the rash was present.

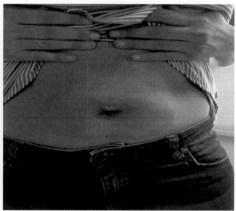

From a tick in the navel.

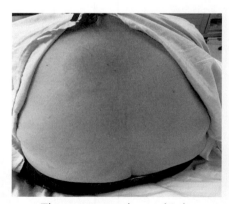

The spots may be multiple.

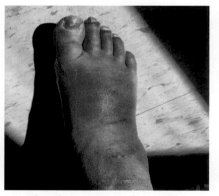

The changes may be subtle.

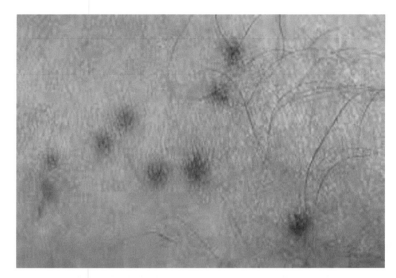

Insect bites, often caused by mosquitos. Small itchy and last 48hrs. These are not associated with Lyme Disease.

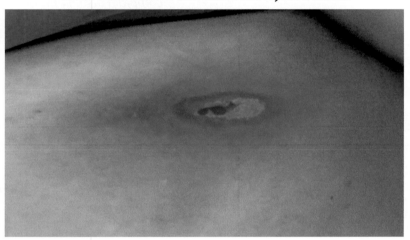

The lesion may break down centrally in less than 5% of cases.

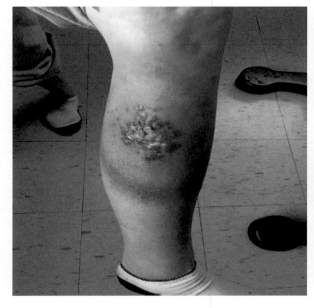

Unusual degree of central breakdown.

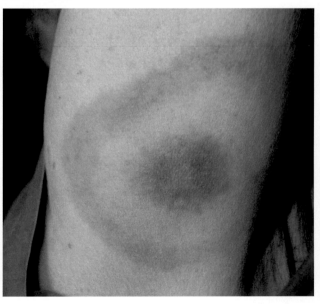

About one in ten DO look like a bullseye, Source: CDC/James Gathany

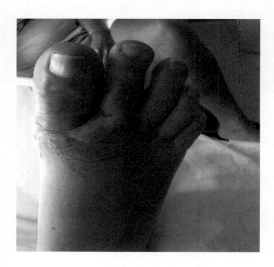

*This man was thought to
have athlete's foot!*

The presence of a flu like illness and a typical rash is diagnostic of acute Lyme disease, which is straightforward in an endemic area such as the Northeastern United States. Treatment with antibiotics should be started. Antibody tests at this time will be negative but can be tested for again at four to eight weeks. They will become positive if it is Lyme disease with or without treatment. Treatment of Acute Lyme is highly successful with over 90% cure of the acute infection with three to four weeks of doxycycline (not to be used in pregnant or lactating women). It used to be said that doxycycline should not be used in children under the age of 8 because it would damage their teeth. Although true of a similar antibiotic, tetracycline, it is not true of doxycycline. You must also warn patients that exposure to the sun while taking doxycycline can lead to severe sunburn.

An alternative is amoxicillin or cefuroxime axetil. Since the overwhelming majority are cured by this treatment most patients do not return for the blood test at four to eight weeks, even if the physician strenuously recommends it. Why go to the doctor if you feel well?

If an infected patient is not treated the acute flu like illness will resolve by itself in seven to ten days. Wellbeing will return and the patient will not be aware that he or she is vulnerable now to the later features of Lyme.

Chapter Two
HOW CAN YOU GET LYME DISEASE AND NOT KNOW IT?

1. You may be infected with *B Burgdorferi* and have no or only mild symptoms. Between five and ten percent of people who develop antibodies to *B burgdorferi*, meaning they definitely have been infected, have no recollection of an acute illness or a spot. Asymptomatic infection undoubtedly occurs.
2. As many as 30% of people with the flu-like illness of acute Lyme disease either have no rash, or miss or misinterpret it. They think they have the flu. A physician will acknowledge that a feverish illness may be due to Lyme, particularly in the summer months, without a rash and have a low threshold for treating such patients with doxycycline, or at the very least will see them again at six weeks to repeat the blood test.
3. You may decline treatment even if you have symptoms and a rash.
4. You may for several reasons take an incomplete course of treatment.

That's a lot of people who have been infected with *Bb* who feel healthy and aren't cured. If you live in an endemic zone this is a good argument for having a yearly Lyme test with your annual checkup.

What happens to you if you are infected and do not know it?

Chapter Three
EARLY DISSEMINATED LYME

There are three stages of Lyme disease.
1. Acute Lyme - described in Chapter 1.
2. Early disseminated disease
3. Late disseminated disease.

The stages overlap.

Features of early disseminated Lyme

Facial Palsy

Case History.

An 8 yr old boy living with his three sisters and a brother on his father's farm developed weakness of his right face developing over an hour and a half. There was neither numbness nor pain. He lost the ability to smile on that side although he could wrinkle his forehead. His mum noted that he had been sick for about a week and she brought him to the doctor because she noticed three big red spots on his back. She also noticed that he was getting weak in his left face too. Tick bites were common where they lived. To get bitten was a normal part of farm life. He was a healthy happy go lucky child always out playing in the yard with his siblings.

On examination the right side of his face was immobile. He could wrinkle his forehead. The left side was also weak although not so bad as the right. On general examination he had three ECMs. Two on his back and one behind his right knee.

Lyme disease is common in children. They play outdoors. Facial palsy, usually affecting one side, is a manifestation of Lyme. If it affects both sides, as it occasionally will, it is *particularly* suggestive of Lyme.

Bell's palsy, i.e., facial palsy of unknown cause, is not rare. It has been attributed to Herpes Simplex Virus infection. There are a few other uncommon causes. But in the Lyme Zone, *Bb* is most frequent.

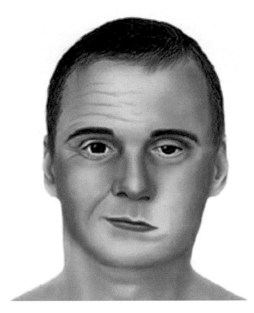

*Artists's impression of paralysis of
the right seventh cranial nerve.
Source: CDC*

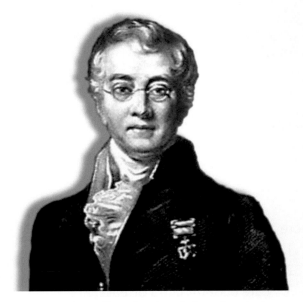

*Sir Charles Bell credited with first description
of paralysis of the seventh cranial nerve.*

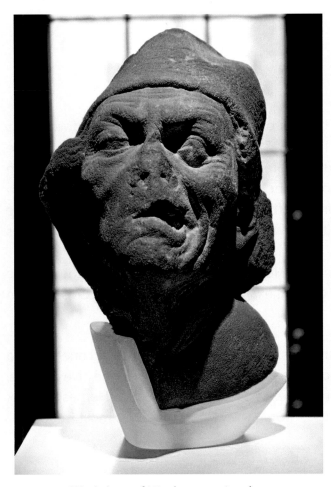

*Workshop of Nicolaus von Leyden.
Head of Man with a Facial Paralysis.
Source: Cancer/Wikimedia Commons*

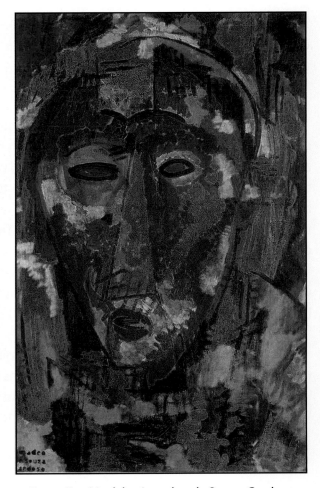

Green Eye Mask by Amadeo de Souza Cordoso.

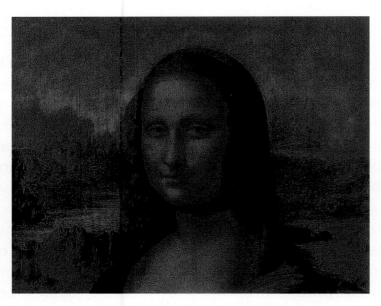

Mona Lisa by Leonardo da Vinci.

Sir Charles Bell (1774-1842), a Scotsman, described it and gave it its name, although as is often the case in the History of Medicine it had been described previously.

It has been argued that since Bell described facial palsy of unknown cause and since in the case of Lyme disease, the cause, *Bb,* is known, facial palsy in Lyme should not be called Bell's palsy.
It should be called, *Borrelia burgdorferi lower motor neurone palsy of the seventh cranial nerve.*
　　Seems like a fine point.
　　Is it possible that the Mona Lisa's enigmatic smile is due to a Bell's palsy? The more I look at the right side of her face the more I think it might be. Do you think she had Lyme disease?

　　Five percent of people infected with *B burgdorferi* will develop Bell's palsy. Sorry, *lower motor neurone paralysis of the seventh cranial nerve due to B burgdorferi.*
　　Other peripheral nerves may be involved. The rare Involvement of the optic nerve and auditory nerve may lead to blindness or deafness. The fifth or trigeminal cranial nerve may be involved leading to a typical kind of facial pain called trigeminal neuralgia. The question is, does it represent infection of the lining of the brain, meningitis, or of the brain itself encephalitis? The seventh, and these other cranial nerves are peripheral, so their involvement does not automatically signify a deeper infection.

Other Eye Involvement

　　The eye is involved in Lyme in a variety of ways, not just optic atrophy. Inflammaatiion can affect any part of the eye with dryness, redness, pain and impaired vision. The technical names for these involvements are iridocyclitis, vitritis, multifocal choriditis, exudative retinal detachment and panophthalmitis. These findings are nonspecific so the physician must maintain his high level of suspicion.

Meningitis

We know from experience that meningitis quite often goes together with Facial Palsy so a spinal tap to prove or dismiss it is frequently performed. If it shows meningitis the treatment is intravenous antibiotics, Ceftriaxone or Penicillin, for three to four weeks.

Meningitis is a terrifying word. We share atavistic memories of an explosive childhood illness, common before antibiotics, with a hundred percent mortality. But Lyme meningitis is *subacute*, remember. It is so laid back that the patient may not even complain of headache and the diagnosis is missed. Don't misunderstand me. This is a real and serious condition, but the terror sometimes associated with the word can be downgraded to appropriate concern.

What's worse, the expression *spinal tap* carries, for the average patient, another layer of dread. It shouldn't. It is extremely safe once raised intracranial pressure is ruled out by clinical examination or Computerized Tomography (CT) scan or both. These days spinal tap is performed with local anesthesia and, often, CT guided needle placement. Meningitis is established by the presence of abnormal numbers of white cells called lymphocytes and the presence of antibodies to *Bb*. Protein levels will be high.

What other Nervous system involvement is seen in early disseminated Lyme disease?

Radiculitis.

The word means infection in the sheath of nerves as they leave the spinal cord.

This is painful. A constant severe aching pain, difficult to describe in the neck or back, made worse by coughing, sneezing or straining.

If a spinal tap is performed the CSF will show the same findings as in meningitis, as there is a local inflammation of the nerve sheath, derived from meninges. Root pain and abnormal CSF due to Lyme, is known as Bannwarth's syndrome after the German clinician who first described it in the nineteen forties. It may be misdiagnosed as prolapsed disc or sciatica which is a disaster as the disease responds well to antibiotics. If it is not treated the swelling will destroy the nerve leading to paralysis.

Acute features of Lyme such as the big red spot, fever, malaise, aches and pains may or may not be present with this syndrome. Lyme tests are positive. Patients do well with antibiotic therapy but badly without. This emphasizes as ever the importance of early diagnosis. Late diagnosis may lead to permanent, irreversible paralysis.

Borrelial Lymphocytoma

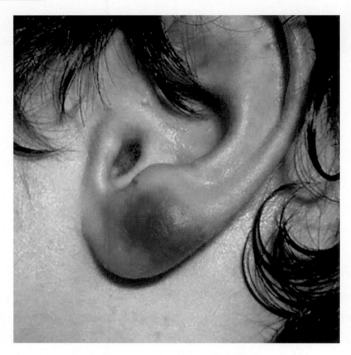

An example of Borrelia lymphocytoma.

Borrelial Lymphocytoma is a painless nodule on the ear lobe or breast. It is found elsewhere on the body rarely. It is more often seen in children than adults. Other features of acute Lyme described in Chapter One may be seen. It responds well to 2 to 4 weeks of antibiotics. Of the 10% that fail to respond a second two-week course usually cures.

Lyme Disease in Pregnancy

Borrelia burgdorferi can cross the placenta and cause death of the fetus or congenital malformations. It is extremely rare for it to do so.

There are no such cases reported in pregnant women who have been treated for Lyme disease acquired during pregnancy.

Treatment is the same as in the non-pregnant except that doxycycline should be avoided.

Typically, amoxicillin 500mgs three times a day for two to four weeks is used. If you are allergic, cefuroxime axetil is an alternative.

Chapter Four
MORE EARLY DISSEMINATED LYME

Cardiac disease

Can you die from Lyme disease?

You can, but only a very few have suffered this misfortune.

The risk of death is entirely restricted to the 1% of infected people who have involvement of the heart. In the USA, 30,000 confirmed cases of Lyme disease are reported. As stated before, the real number will be much higher. Of those 30,000, 2,000 people a year will have an infected heart. From 1985 to 2019 there have been 11 reported deaths.

Rare or not, and making allowances for considerable under reporting, we are talking about a curable disease and therefore we should always be thinking of the possibility. When patients complain of breathlessness, palpitations, dizziness, fainting, or chest pain, consider Lyme. Doctors call this having a high index of suspicion. For Lyme carditis it can't be too high.

Case History.

A 29-year-old otherwise healthy policeman

fell to the ground while on duty at the station. He was taken to the Emergency Room of the local hospital. He had lost consciousness but was coming round on arrival. He had a heart rate of 36 per minute, normal being 60-90 beats per minute. EKG showed complete heart block which means that the usual connection between the upper and lower chambers of the heart is blocked in this case by infection. Luckily the ventricles beat by themselves but at a low rate predisposing the patient to fall to the ground. This is called a Stokes-Adams attack.

There are a number of possible causes of heart block, but in the Lyme Zone, *Bb* is the commonest. The patient was taken to the intensive care unit and his heart rate monitored. He was restored and uncomplaining without other relevant history. There were no abnormal findings on exam except for his slow heart rate. His two-tier Lyme antibody test came back strongly positive. Since he was so well and under medical supervision it was decided not to place an artificial pacemaker but to treat him with intravenous Ceftriaxone. The next morning his heart was back in normal rhythm.

Not every patient responds so promptly and there is a role for a temporary pacemaker although many will resolve on antibiotics alone.

Lyme can also cause other abnormal rhythms of heart beat and rarely weakness of the heart muscle itself. It is this, myocarditis, which can be lethal. An evaluation of the eleven reported deaths noted that delay in diagnosis was a significant part of the poor outcome.

Arthritis.

8% of people infected with Lyme get arthritis.

Lyme causes arthritis which means swelling, pain, and reduced range of movement of a joint. Lyme affects large weight bearing joints one at a time, usually, the commonest being the knee. It typically occurs between one and four months after the original infection and it ranges from a mild disease that responds rapidly to antibiotic therapy to a severe persistent antibiotic refractory swollen, painful joint.

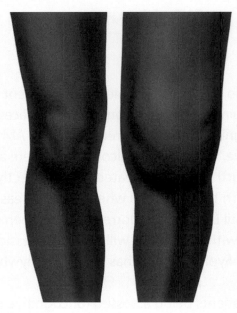

Early diagnosis is essential. When neglected it can lead to permanent joint damage.
Source: CDC

Treatment is four weeks of oral antibiotics. It is very effective, yet it does not cure everybody.

How many doesn't it cure and why not?

About 20% are not cured and their arthritis gets worse despite treatment. This is called post-infectious Lyme arthritis. Since you ask, it is caused by high amounts of gamma interferon and low amounts of the anti-inflammatory interleukin 10. This leads to impaired tissue repair, vascular damage, cytotoxic autoimmune processes, fibroblast proliferations and fibrosis.

To put it another way, the immune response is out of whack. Why some people should get it and others not, is unknown. Of interest to future researchers, these changes look very like Rheumatoid arthritis under the microscope.

Here we see undoubted evidence of immunologic damage to the joint in addition to the direct, harmful effects of infection.

Chapter Five
<u>LATE DISSEMINATED LYME</u>

As life expectancy increases so dementia becomes more frequent. One in seven Americans over the age of 70 has evidence of forgetfulness, disorientation in familiar places, loss of recent memory and other mental stigmata of impaired cognition. The top three causes are Alzheimer's disease, multiple strokes (vascular dementia) and excessive, longstanding alcohol use. There are several less-common causes.

Wait a minute. There is a fourth. Lyme, untreated or imperfectly treated. *Bb* gets into the brain. So, if you live in the North Eastern United States where Lyme disease is hyperendemic, no diagnosis of dementia can be accepted until Lyme, neuroborreliosis, has been excluded. This is most important as it can be treated. Treatment with antibiotics will stop progression of the disease. This is entirely reminiscent of our knowledge of Syphilis. Which has not gone anywhere and *also* needs exclusion. I'm going to put it in red capitals, EARLY DIAGNOSIS IS ESSENTIAL.

In a review in our office of patients being assessed for cognitive impairment, including spinal tap, 30 out of 90 subjects had positive antibody tests for Lyme in the CSF, thus proving neurolyme. 27 had positive tests in the blood. Blood tests, therefore, are a good screening test, but if your suspicion is high and the patient is relatively healthy spinal tap must be performed even if serum antibodies are negative.

Researchers have examined the hypothesis that Lyme infection causes Alzheimer's disease and/or other chronic neurological disorders such as Multiple Sclerosis, Lou Gehrig's disease and Lewy body dementia but no evidence supporting these hypotheses has been found.

Case History

A 44-year-old mother of two was brought by her family for evaluation as she was making elementary mathematical errors in her job as a superintendent at a supermarket. What worried them most was her inappropriate behavior. She had changed over the last year from the responsible worker she had been to a giggling, unfocussed mistake-making, forgetful person.

She had moved to the area in the mid-Hudson valley about three years ago having previously lived in New York City. For about fifteen years, between the ages of 15 to 30 she would come to the area as her family had a weekend house near the Ashokan reservoir. They loved to go for long walks through the woodlands of the Catskills.

Both blood and cerebrospinal fluid showed the presence of many antibody bands to Bb. She was treated with intravenous antibiotics for a month with minor improvement.

Treatment with intravenous Ceftriaxone for four weeks will prevent progression of the disease.

Acrodermatitis chronicum atrophicans (ACA)

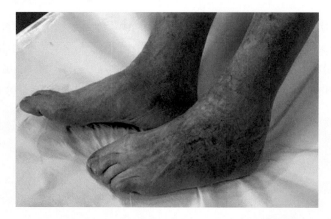

Acrodermatitis chronica atroficans (ACA)

This manifestation of Lyme disease is said to be commoner in the European version of the disease, mostly caused by *Borrelia afzeli*, but it certainly can be found west of the Atlantic. This is probably the most underdiagnosed manifestation of Lyme. It is an irregular discoloration of the skin usually seen on the legs and as its name suggests lasts for a long time. In some patients there are recurrent effusions in the local joints and damage to the local nerves. Some have severe localized pain. Some present with the exhaustion syndrome and some have cognitive impairment, so this skin lesion is much more than an interesting observation.

It will respond to antibiotic therapy albeit slowly.

Post Treatment Lyme Disease Syndrome, PTLDS

After adequate treatment for Acute Lyme a minority of patients become easily exhausted, have sleep disturbance, brain fog, aches and pains in the muscles and joints, and their quality of life is markedly impaired.

How many exactly? The literature gives contradictory views from 0% to 80%. The best study, from Johns Hopkins University, says 14% in the strict conditions of a research study and notes that the number in the "real world" is likely to be higher because of misdiagnosis and delay in treatment. In the absence of specific markers of the disease, it becomes a diagnosis of exclusion. There is no doubt as to the existence of the syndrome, but from my experience, I am am surprised it is as high as 15% but I accept this figure. It is commoner after treatment for late features of the disease and about two thirds of the sufferers have underlying chronic ailments such as diabetes and rheumatoid arthritis.

There is much debate as to the cause of this exhaustion, this prolonged convalescence, this Long Lyme. It will be discussed in more detail in the chapters which follow.

Cutaneous B-cell lymphoma

This rare form of cancer of the skin has been associated with *Borrelia burgdorferi.* For years this association was only observed in Europe, and was attributed to *Borrelia afzeli* the predominant European strain. More recent studies have shown a correlation in the USA with Bb. The association of a bacterial infection with skin cancer is highly significant and there are case reports of this tumor responding to antibiotics.

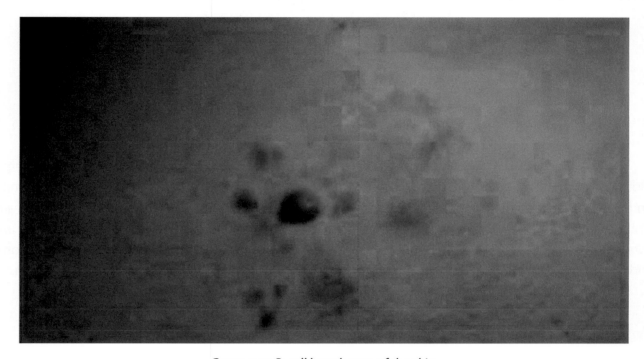

Cuteneous B-cell lymphoma of the skin.

Loose association with a large number of diseases have been reported including Morphoea, Perry-Romberg Syndrome, Lou Gehrig disease and Multiple Sclerosis.

Can infection with *Borrelia burgdorferi* be the cause of, or an exacerbating factor, of other illnesses? Particularly rare illnesses of unknown cause? To date, the evidence is inconclusive.

To take the last example, Multiple Sclerosis (MS); neuro Lyme can certainly mimic MS, but they are separate diseases not least because neuro Lyme may respond to antibiotic therapy. Further research is underway.

Chapter Six
CO-INFECTIONS

American Ticks transmit 17 disease causing organisms. Others are likely to be discovered.
Can you acquire more than one infection at a time?
Yes.
Case history
High fever, confusion and a paralyzed right arm in a 55-year-old IBM worker who has taken early retirement on grounds of ill health.

The patient presented with delirium.
He could not answer simple direct questions.
On examination his temperature was 40 degrees Centigrade, his right arm hung limply by his side being weak and wasted.
His neck was slightly stiff raising the possibility of meningitis. He was mildly jaundiced. He had no skin lesions of Lyme disease.

His blood work was abnormal across the board. He had a low white cell count, a low platelet count, abnormal liver function tests, with a slightly elevated bilirubin. His kidney function was at the upper limit of normal. CXR and CT scan were within normal limits although the CT scan of his brain showed nonspecific linear opacities. Urine was positive for urobilinogen which suggests breakdown of the red blood cells. He was transferred to the ICU and treated empirically with intravenous doxycycline, azithromycin and atovaquone. A spinal tap was performed and showed an abnormal number of white blood cells, 96, of which 90% were lymphocytes. The protein was elevated and the glucose level was slightly low.

Ceftriaxone was added to the antibiotic regimen.

His wife told his remarkable story.

Her husband's father had migrated from Italy after World War two and worked in construction. He was an avid hunter and when his son, the patient (H) was a teenager, he took him into the woods. H killed his first deer at the age of 16 and he continued to hunt until his mid-twenties when he had an epiphany and gave up hunting on the principle that he should be kind to living things. He became a supporter of deer, leaving food for them in his yard. About five years before this admission, he developed severe pain in his right arm. The pain was constant and made worse by coughing or sneezing. The diagnosis was pinched nerve. He saw a number of doctors including orthopedists who could not find anything to operate on. Gradually he lost power in that arm, the muscles wasted away and the pain slowly abated.

His positive attitude to deer continued and a number would come to his yard every morning and over a season he got to recognize them and apparently, they him. He took photos of himself with his arm round a living deer. They would gather and he would feed them. He was bitten by ticks, and had devised ways of removing them.

With the assistance of specific laboratory tests the following diagnoses were made.

1. Lyme meningitis
2. Anaplasmosis
3. Babesiosis
4. Lyme radiculopathy

He had a full house.

This patient made an excellent recovery except for his arm. He was treated for four weeks for his meningitis with intravenous ceftriaxone. He did not develop prolonged convalescence or PTLDS.

Where I practice, about a hundred miles north of New York City, by the banks of the sweet-flowing Hudson, there are three common microbes that may be transmitted singly or in combination from tick bite. The first is Lyme disease.
The other two are Anaplasmosis and Babesiosis.
50% of the blacklegged ixodes tick carry Bb for starters. From 5 to 12 % of patients with acute Lyme have a second infection with one of these two organisms.
About 1% have all three.
Another patient of mine with all three organisms *did* suffer a prolonged convalescence with exhaustion, pains and clicking in his joints, sleep disturbance and brain fog. After a year he had improved but was only about sixty percent better. With the support of his wife and family and without further antibiotics he returned to his baseline at 18 months.

Anaplasmosis.

Its name means "without shape".
It is a *rickettsial* organism, a group of bacteria the first of which was discovered by the Ohio physician Howard Ricketts as the cause of Rocky Mountain Spotted Fever in 1906.
They live primarily in insects such as lice, mosquitoes and ticks and cause an array of acute infections in humans.
Anaplasmosis causes sudden onset of high fever with shaking chills and rigors. Aches and pains in muscles and joints are frequently experienced as with most feverish illnesses. Rash may be seen in ten percent of patients. Their bloodwork is typical with a low white blood cell count, a low platelet count and abnormal liver function tests of mild to moderate degree. It occurs in six percent of patients with acute Lyme, (range 2-12%).
The infection responds rapidly to doxycycline.
Similar rickettsiae in the family Ehrlichia are transmitted mainly by the Lone Star Tick, which does

occur in the north east but is more usually found in the southeastern US states, including Texas. They cause an identical disease.

Babesiosis

Babesia microti is named after the Hungarian vet Victor Babes who discovered it as the cause of an epidemic in cattle in 1888. It is a *protozoa* or single celled organism like malaria or amebiasis. It is a *piroplasma,* to be precise, which means a protozoa transmitted to animals, including humans by a tick. The first description in humans was in Yugoslavia in 1957. The first case in the USA was in California in 1966. In 1968 a man who had previously had a splenectomy died from babesiosis on Fire island, New York. It was erroneously thought, for a few years, only to cause disease in humans without spleens i.e., "this man can't have babesiosis, he has an intact spleen." Medicine progresses slowly in this way, learning as we go, a dogma-revising process.

Patients often present with abrupt onset of high fever which is reminiscent of Anaplasmosis and the distinction can only be made by blood tests. Since the microorganism lives in red blood cells and breaks them up (hemolysis), patients may become anemic and have features of hemolysis, the simplest sign of which is mild jaundice and the presence of urobilinogen in the urine. There are other confirmatory tests of hemolysis, but these findings would be sufficient to warrant starting specific anti-babesia antibiotics the commonest used of which are Azithromycin and Atovaquone the latter being a well-known anti-malarial.

Babesiosis may rarely cause life threatening infection. Curiously there may also be no symptoms at all, but most often there is a febrile illness with good response to treatment. Does it recur? It may recur once, rarely twice if untreated, particularly in immunocompromised patients. Each subsequent attack is milder than the one before.

This protozoa and in its microbiology and the disease it causes has earned it at least one nickname, Malaria of the Hudson Valley.

These are the three main co-infections with Lyme. Protective immunity against these infections is weak and it is possible to be infected several times.

Coinfections with a number of other agents may more rarely occur
Borrelia mayoni. A disease found mainly in the upper Midwest of the United States. This tick transmitted bacteria causes a disease that is similar to Lyme with an increased tendency to nausea and vomiting and larger more diffuse rashes.

Borrelia miyamotoi. More widely distributed than *mayoni* it is seen in the north-east and leads to a disease indistinguishable clinically from acute Lyme disease due to *Borrelia burgdorferi*.

It was first discovered in Japan in 1995, further testimony to *Borrelia's* cosmopolitan nature.

Powassan

A number of viruses are rarely transmitted by ticks particularly, *Powassan* a flavivirus. It is named after a town in Ontario and means "bend in the river" in first nation language. The infection may range from asymptomatic to life threatening inflammation of the lining of the brain or the brain itself called meningoencephalitis.It was first described in 2008 and each year since. Less than 20 cases are reported yearly in the USA. Making allowances for underreporting it is still a rare disease. There are a handful of case reports of co-infection with Lyme.

Other rare infectious agents transmitted by ticks include *Bourbon* virus, Tularemia, Tick borne relapsing fever (*Borrelia hermsii, Borrelia turicate*) Rocky Mountain Spotted Fever (rarely seen in the Rocky Mountains), *Rickettsia parkeri* and *ehrlichia muris eauclairensis*

Bartonella

This family of gram negative bacteria has 22 species, 14 of which are known, to date, to cause disease in humans. It deserves a book in its own right. It occurs in many animals, including domesticated cats and dogs. The best-known infection caused by bartonella in the USA is cat-scratch fever. These organisms are transmitted to humans by the bites of "vectors", from sandflies, lice, fleas and *ticks*.

The question is, is it a co-infection? There are several case reports of people infected with Lyme and bartonella and it exists in Ixodes ticks. Yet there is no direct evidence that it is transmitted to humans by ticks. Epidemiological studies show no difference in the incidence of Bartonella in patients with Lyme disease and those without.

Given its ubiquity and its ability to cause the exhaustion syndrome in its own right it is entirely reasonable to look for it by means of antibody testing should the patient have difficult to treat symptoms, particularly if their immune system is compromised. It has been suggested that it may be responsible for PTLDS which is a hypothesis awaiting confirmation.

Mycoplasma

These are the smallest bacteria. They are a common cause of mild or "walking" pneumonia and otitis media. They have been discovered in ticks but there is no evidence that they are transmitted to humans by biting insects.

M. fermentans is the smallest of all organisms in this family of small bacteria. Several large-scale studies have failed to show disease in humans after infection with this organism.

Part Two
LYME AND THE EXHAUSTION SYNDROME

Chapter Seven
THE EXHAUSTION SYNDROME.

'Doctor, I'm tired all the time.'
This is one of the commonest complaints a patient will bring to my office as an infectious disease specialist.
'I have poor sleep/pains in the muscles and the joints/irritability/dizziness/can't sleep/ despondency/ / headache/always tired/
I used to be full of life always active. Now I don't want to do anything. Something is medically wrong with me.'

A collection of symptoms like this is common amongst humans living in developed city centred societies in the 21st century.
Clearly these patients are unwell. Come on now Mr. Doctor Doctor, figure out why.

First, I accept these patients at face value. They are not making their symptoms up.

This is true even in the absence of objective evidence of disease. The exhaustion syndrome is common, and we don't understand the underlying pathology, and we don't understand what causes the actual symptoms; exhaustion, joint pain, muscle pain, sleep disturbance, malaise, brain fog. The history of Medicine is littered with illnesses from tuberculosis to tinnitus that have been blamed on the patient until the actual cause was found. It has never once been the patient's fault, so why should it be so in this case?
Although the mechanism of the syndrome, its *biochemistry* is unknown in many cases, we have learned how to evaluate such patients and offer valid advice.

Can Lyme present this way?
Yes.
1. Prolonged convalescence after acute Lyme.
2. Post Treatment Lyme Disease Syndrome. There is an overlap between one and two.
3. As a manifestation of undiagnosed Lyme.

Therefore, if you work in the Lyme zone you will be alert to these possibilities.
However, there are at least thirty other causes to be considered (see table).
Missing the diagnosis of Lyme disease is a serious error; diagnosing Lyme when the symptoms are caused by another disease is equally so.

Case History.

A 65-year-old retired hospital administrator

complains of exhaustion. He sleeps late. When he gets out of bed, he feels tired. Every little project is arduous. He sleeps in the afternoon. He often has a throbbing headache, pain in his left shoulder and dizziness on exertion.

His appetite is poor, and he has lost eight pounds in weight over the last six months which coincides with the period of time he has felt exhausted.

He lives in the mid-Hudson valley and plays golf, although he hasn't been able to find the energy to do this recently. He is depressed.

He has a wife and three healthy children. He neither smokes nor drinks.

His wife is convinced he has Lyme disease and is urging early treatment with antibiotics. The physician agrees it is possible but urges her to let him examine her husband and to do some blood tests and X-rays.

On examination the physician finds thickening of an artery on one side of his head and no other abnormality. He orders tests and arranges for a biopsy of the thickened artery.

"In the meantime," he advises, "stay hydrated, take vitamins, and take it easy. I'll see you in three days."

"Why not order the antibiotics now so that we can start them as soon as possible?" asked his wife.

"We haven't made a diagnosis yet."

"You mean you don't think he has Lyme? I know he has Lyme because I'm his wife, and I have researched it online. If we don't give him antibiotics within twenty-four hours, I'm going to take him to a Lyme literate doctor."

He had the tiny artery in his forehead biopsied under local anesthesia as an outpatient. The next evening, he is brought to the emergency room because of chest pain suggestive of a heart attack. He is admitted and this is ruled out. He complains of constant pain in his left chest and shoulder. Some tests are back. He has a mild anemia, an ESR of 98 mms in the first hour, (abnormally high), negative screening test for Lyme antibodies.

His chest Xray is normal.

His wife insists he be treated for Lyme disease with antibiotics.

"What is there to lose?" she enquires angrily. She lodges a complaint with the hospital administration and informs the doctor she has written a letter of complaint to the State Medical Board. She insists on a second opinion which the physician is happy to provide. He recommends and arranges transfer of the patient to the Medical Center by ambulance.

Two days later the biopsy report shows vasculitis, a disease called Giant Cell arteritis which explains his symptoms. It is not a rare disease. Follow up western blot Lyme test is repeatedly negative.

He is put on methyl prednisolone by mouth in a high dose and his symptoms improve.

Two weeks later he is in fine form. All his symptoms have resolved, and the dose of steroids is being slowly tapered down.

Of a hundred patients presenting with the Exhaustion Syndrome;

Fifteen percent will have a diagnosable organic disease (see table).

Five percent will have primary depression or bipolar disorder.

If you have the exhaustion syndrome you might get secondarily depressed which makes you more tired in a vicious cycle. The five percent I mention here refers to primary psychiatric disorder.

Thirty percent will have prolonged convalescence with a diagnosed infectious agent. This group has an excellent prognosis for complete recovery, with supportive care, that may take from six months to two years.

Thirty percent will have prolonged convalescence without a diagnosed infectious agent. The history may be suggestive. This group has a less good outcome.

Twenty five percent will continue to be exhausted and no cause is found.

An incomplete list of the causes of Exhaustion.

Anemia:	Iron deficiency (heavy periods, slow loss of blood into the intestines, other causes.)
Other Hematological disease:	Lymphoma
	Myeloma
	Chronic leukemia
Psychiatric illness	Depressioin "Noonday demon"
	Bipolar disease
Endocrine disease	Hypothyrodiism
	Hypoadrenalism (Addison's disease)
	Hyperparathyroidism
	Impaired testicular function
	Menopause
Vitamin D deficiency	
Prolonged Convalescence	Exhaustion syndrome after acute iinfectious illness
	Post Mono syndrome
	Post Viral syndrome
	Long Covid
	Post-Influenza
	Post-Lyme disease
	Post treatment Lyme disease
	Post-any acute infection
	Post major surgery

Undiagnosed Chronic Infections	Human Immunodeficiency Virus
	Hepatitis C Virus
	Brucellosis
	Cytomegalovirus
	Epstein-Barr Virus
	Toxoplasmosis
	Human herpes virus 6
	Qfever
	Bartonellosis
	Lyme disease
Rheumatological disease	Systemic Lupus Erythematosis
	Rheumatoid arthritis
	Polymyalgia rheumatica
	Vasculitis
	Fibromyalgia
Drugs or Medicines	Antihistamines
	Antidepressants; such as amitriptyline (Elavil)
	Anxiety medicines; such as lorazepam (Ativan)
	Antihypertensives; Beta blockers such as metoprolol
	Chemotherapy
	Anticonvulsants; such as phenytoin (Dilantin)
	Cholesteral lowering agents; such as statins
Other	Postural tachycardia syndrome (PoTS)
	Adult onset Mitochondrial disorder
	Gulf War Syndrome
	Post-traumatic stress disorder

Chapter Eight
A HISTORY OF EXHAUSTION

The Exhaustion syndrome is the nonspecific response of the body to a large number of possible causes, some of which are unknown and one of which is Lyme disease.

In our contemporary world it is often attributed to *stress,* to *burnout,* often with *brainfog.* Yet its history suggests it has always afflicted mankind.

Hippocrates described it two thousand years ago.

A few hundred years later, Galen is reinforcing his teaching; "exhaustion is caused by a surplus of black bile. The body tries to burn it, but the dust rises from the stomach to the brain and clouds vision of the world."

St John Chrysostom, the archbishop of Constantinople, wrote in the fifth century, *Qui febri laborat, post morbum infirmior est.* He who suffers a fever is weaker after the illness.

Moses ben Maimon also known as Maimonides and Rambam (1135-1204) the philosopher, jurist and pre-eminent physician of the middle ages even had a treatment for the exhaustion syndrome. ....*one may rid himself of it by listening to singing and all kinds of instrumental music, by strolling through beautiful gardens and splendid buildings, by gazing upon beautiful pictures and other things that enliven the mind and dissipate gloomy moods. The purpose of all this is to restore the healthy condition of the body, but the real object in maintaining the body in good health is to acquire wisdom.*

Acedia or Accedie, (acciditties in middle English).

Variously defined as sadness, listlessness, not caring, laziness, hopelessness. It afflicted monks and was distressing in the extreme. The monk cannot concentrate, cannot study, he is always tired, "he looks at the sun as if it were too slow in setting"

The abbot Evagrius of Pontus in the late fourth century called it the most troublesome of all the evil thoughts. It poisons the mind with discontent and is the action of a demon. He urges constant vigilance against this "vice" that is the container of other vices. This noonday demon "envelops the entire soul and strangles the mind".

He would counsel sufferers and is therefore the first documented psychotherapist.

Dante Alighieri wrote The Divine Comedy when he was 35 in response to feeling "lost in a dark wood."

He writes that *underneath the water there are souls who sigh: we are bitter in the blackened mud."*

Sloth

Sloth is similar to acedia but could be applied to anyone, not just monks. It is one of the seven deadly sins, namely: Pride, Greed, Lust, Envy, Gluttony, Wrath and Sloth.

Sloth: boredom, rancor, apathy, inert sluggish mentation, sleep disturbance, indifference to work, 'laziness.' (Snap out of it or you'll go to hell).

Melancholy. means black bile.

Robert Burton wrote The Anatomy of Melancholy, first published in 1621. He describes
A kind of dotage without a fever, having for his ordinary companions, fear and sadness without any apparent occasion.

Shakespeare's entire cannon is infused with ideas of melancholy and raises the question, is it an illness or an integral part of the human psyche? Jacques in As You Like It is known as Monsieur Melancholy. He says, "I do love it better than laughing."

Slow recovery from Typhus

Dr Gerard Boate, physician to Oliver Cromwell wrote in 1650: *"(typhus) occurs with great violence, that notwithstanding all good helps, some are thereby carried to their graves; and others who come off with their lives are forced to keep to their beds a long time from extreme weakness."*

Sexual Impropriety.

Fast forward to Victorian times where in a significant shift, masturbation, infidelity, reading pornography were the cause of exhaustion and listlessness.

Convalescence.

It is difficult for us to imagine life in the cities of Europe and the World before the discovery of the existence of bacteria and viruses and their causative role in the abundant scourges of the time. We take antibiotics and vaccines for granted. Man's normal state was to live in a sink of infectious diseases with unexpected death pending at any moment. Tuberculosis, typhoid, cholera, typhus, dysentery, syphilis, measles, influenza, to name but the worst, could afflict you and carry you off at any moment.

The word convalescence came to the fore in late nineteenth century Europe and was the beginning of contemporary thought on the problem.

CONVALESCENCE. CON... with; VALESCERE; to grow strong, your state of gradual return to health after illness, a gentle process of recovery. Most of us have experienced it. You've got Flu, the worst is over. You have no fever; your cough is better. The headache's gone. But you remain tired, listless and apathetic. Over the next few days to a week that washed out feeling fades away and you are back to your normal self. The hurricane has passed, now we must rebuild what is damaged.

In some people, and we don't know why, convalescence may persist from six months to two years and, rarely, longer.

In Victorian times it was mainly a luxury for the rich to travel to spa towns, mountain and seaside resorts. Reformers and philanthropists, however, built homes away from the cities for the poor. Florence Nightingale was a strong advocate. Fresh air and a nutritious diet were the mainstay of convalescent support.

Neurasthenia

The American neurologist George Beard renamed the exhaustion syndrome *neurasthenia* in 1862. It was attributed to too much brainwork. Only the sensitive, creative and refined could suffer from it. It took off like a rocket. Anyone who was anyone had neurasthenia. It was not for the lower classes, however, or for non-American, non-European peoples. In other words, it became a means of reinforcing prejudice. In 1874 the psychiatrist, Henry Maudsley, taught that we have limited energy and women's is all concentrated in their reproductive organs. Squandering it on writing and studying would hurt them. Women who worked would suffer terrible physical consequences. Yes, prejudices can be medicalized.

Towards the end of the nineteenth century exhaustion was being blamed on trains, the telegraph, the pace of modern life, information overload. Sigmund Freud said that the cause of mal-aise was civilization itself. We did not evolve to get on public transport and go to an office. The ego, the super-ego and the id are in a constant battle. It takes energy to repress our desires.

As medical science began to characterize mental illness, neurasthenia as a concept lost popularity as to have it was to imply you were crazy.

Spanish Influenza

It is estimated that 80 million people died of Spanish influenza. If the mortality was ten percent, then 800 million people were infected with the disease. Prolonged convalescence was common after this infection which led to economic and political disaster. Planting failed in parts of Africa because of widespread inability to work, followed by famine. We have seen for ourselves in the Covid 19 epidemic that plagues bring economic and societal changes along with their typical fevers.

Myalgic Encephalomyelitis (ME)

In 1955 at the Royal Free Hospital in London 292 members of the medical, nursing, auxiliary and administrative staff fell ill with low grade fever, swelling of the lymph nodes, aches and pains. This illness was consistent with a viral infection although no virus was ever identified. About a third of those afflicted suffered from a prolonged convalescence. It was called Myalgic Encephalomyelitis or ME and you can't get more medical than that. Thereafter, people suffering from the Exhaustion syndrome could be told they were suffering from ME. This diagnosis existed only in the UK until about 2010 when it crossed the Atlantic and is now widely used around the world to describe the Exhaustion syndrome. There are no characteristic blood tests with which to diagnose it.

Outbreaks similar to Royal Free disease are not uncommon. Examples are Icelandic disease, (Akureyri disease) Epidemic neuromyasthenia, poliomyelitis-like illness, post-viral fatigue syndrome.

Chronic Fatigue Syndrome

In March 1964, Anthony Epstein, Yvonne Barr and Burt Achong published a paper demonstrating a virus in the tissue of a cancer from Africa called Burkitt's lymphoma. It was named the Epstein Barr Virus (EBV).

A lab technician working in this group acquired Infectious Mononucleosis a well-recognized disease of teenagers and young adults. Further studies showed that 85% of young adults with this disease, "mono," or glandular fever as it is called in the UK, were infected with EBV. A certain percentage, perhaps ten percent of those infected with this syndrome, developed prolonged convalescence or chronic fatigue syndrome.

It was thought for some years that the Exhaustion syndrome, not otherwise diagnosable, was due to infection with EBV. The test is positive in every case.

And here we see the importance of performing control studies. It turns out that EBV is one of the most successful viruses to infect humans. 95% of us have been infected with EBV by age thirty. Only 10% of those people suffer chronic fatigue. Candida, brucellosis and Xenotropic murine leukemia virus-related virus all had a spell of popularity. There is such a thing as fashion in infectious disease.

Cytomegalovirus (CMV), Human immunodeficiency virus (HIV), Toxoplasmosis, Human herpes virus 6 (HHV6) also cause Mono with a similar 10-15% progression to the Chronic Fatigue Syndrome.

Dengue, Chikungunya, West Nile Virus, Ebola, Q Fever, Influenza, Zika may be followed by prolonged convalescence and quite certainly other undiagnosed infections, bacterial or viral.

Long Covid

Readers of this chapter will not be surprised to learn that Covid 19 infection was complicated by prolonged convalescence, called Long Covid. It has all the features of and indeed is a Post Viral syndrome. Yes, certainly, different viruses produce slightly different prolonged convalescences, but all have marked fatigue at the core. There is a long list of other symptoms.

Although Long Covid represents prolonged convalescence, an entity known to the medical profession for two thousand years it has stimulated research in ways previous forms of prolonged convalescence have not. Government funded research is underway on both sides of the Atlantic and elsewhere in the world. Several promising hypotheses have been suggested; persisting reservoirs of SARS-CoV-2 in the tissues, immune dysregulation, reactivation of herpesviruses such as EBV, HHV6, and others, autoimmunity, impact on the microbiome, that is the bacteria that live in a normal human, molecular mimicry, microvascular blood clotting with dysfunction of the lining cells of blood vessels, dysfunctional signaling in the brainstem and /or vagus nerve.

Ten percent of people with Covid 19 infection develop Long Covid.

A third were perfectly healthy before the infection. The other two thirds have a wide range of associative factors including female sex, diabetes, lower income and almost any chronic ill health.

It is not related to the severity of the acute infection.

Chronic Lyme. Post Treatment Lyme Disease Syndrome

Which brings us to the topic of this book. What are these two entities other than prolonged convalescence following an acute infection? It is not unique. Lyme is not the only infectious disease. It is to be expected.
It is Long Lyme.

So, what is the Exhaustion syndrome due to?

Black bile? Sloth? Neurasthenia? Myalgic Encephalomyelitis? Chronic Lyme?
Leading scientific hypotheses to date are that there is
Viral persistence
Chronic inflammation

Autonomic dysfunction
Elevated interferons
Blocked absorption of Tryptophan.
Vagal nerve impairment

But the most interesting work to date comes from researchers at the University of Pennsylvania who suggest that serotonin reduction is the cause of Long Covid triggered by remnants of the virus lingering in the gut.

Serotonin is a neurotransmitter that acts as a hormone. It influences learning, memory, happiness, regulates body temperature, sleep, sexual behavior and hunger.
90% is found in cells lining the GI tract and 10% is in your brain.
In Long Covid, there are persistently low levels of Serotonin that could particularly explain neurological, cognitive and memory problems.
It's relevance to Long Lyme and other forms of the exhaustion syndrome remains to be seen.

Chapter Nine
"YOU HAVEN'T GOT LYME." ACTUALLY, YOU DO.

Do doctors fail to make the diagnosis of Lyme disease when that's what the patient has?

Um, let me see, ah…………

I regret to say that it could happen. Doctors make mistakes.

In her book The Widening Circle, Polly Murray, describes how she, her husband and her four children, living in Lyme Connecticut, had symptoms of fever, arthritis, tiredness and aches and pains.

The book begins with a modestly stated yet devastating critique of physicians. Not only don't they listen they jump to conclusions. If they don't understand your symptoms, they say it's all in your head. They are dismissive. She reports how a doctor said to her, "You know, Mrs. Murray, sometimes people subconsciously *want* to be sick."

She refused to accept that she wasn't ill. She did not want to be sick. She saw ten, perhaps fifteen physicians before she met a rheumatologist, Dr Allen Steere, who listened. He took her complaints seriously and wanted to help her. In 1975, he published a report of 51 people in Lyme with a characteristic *disease*. Dr Steere gave it the name of the town in which Polly Murray and her family lived. When tests were developed, she was positive.

Amy Tan has a story to tell. No one has written more poignantly, more explicitly, more cogently about the failures of some members of the medical profession than Amy Tan the international best seller writer, particularly well known for her first novel, The Joy Luck Club.

She describes how she developed a rash on her ankle followed by a flu like illness when attending a wedding in Dutchess County, New York about a hundred miles from New York City and five miles from my office. Without seeing anyone local, i.e., me, she flew back to California and went to see some likeable, top-notch doctors at a medical center.

They told her she couldn't have Lyme because the rash wasn't a bulls-eye. That the disease didn't exist in California, but because she asked, they would do a blood test. The Lyme test was negative so they told her that that ruled the disease out. The test was not repeated. She worsened over the next two years with an array of terrifying neurological symptoms up to and including hallucinations. (I wonder if Lyme gets mis-diagnosed as schizophrenia?)

She was re-investigated with an array of tests including an antibody test for syphilis but not Lyme.

She writes a mortifying sentence,

"Wait. He thought I was more likely to have Syphilis than Lyme?"

If only she had come to see me or one of my colleagues across the river.

Then she saw a "Lyme literate doctor" who repeated the Lyme test. It came back positive. Having diagnosed her correctly, he treated her with antibiotics with gradual improvement and cure.

Her account of how this disease affected her is to be found on her website. It should be required reading for medical students and doctors.

Dr Neal Spector graduated from medical school in New Jersey in 1982 and became an eminent oncologist. He worked in Massachusetts and ran marathons there through the woods. He began to complain of fatigue that became extreme. He also had a burning sensation in the feet, night terrors, insomnia and weight loss. He experienced rapid beating of the heart. It was a misfortune that by now he was working in Florida. The doctors there had little or no knowledge of Lyme because of its local rareness, like California. For four years he was told that his symptoms were due to "stress". When it became apparent that he had heart disease, and he was told that, he asked "why, then, do I feel so tired?" The doctor replied, "Yes denial is the usual response when patients are told they have heart disease."

He developed complete heart block and the diagnosis of Lyme disease was finally made. He responded well to antibiotics except that his heart had been badly damaged. He underwent transplantation in 2009 and lived on in excellent health for another eleven years dying age 63.

On behalf of the medical profession, I apologize unreservedly to Polly Murray, Amy Tan, Neal Spector and everyone else whose Lyme disease has been misdiagnosed and mistreated.

It is mistakes of this kind that drive patients into the arms of alternative doctors and Quacks.

We must listen. The number of patients with Lyme disease is increasing every year. The tick, *Ixodes scapularis* has undergone a population explosion in the last 20 years. Cases are found across the United States. Cases have been diagnosed in every state of the Union including California and Florida. The incidence is rising in Southern Canada.

We have to listen and most of us do. What's the difference between a good doctor and a bad one? "He or she wouldn't listen to me."

Yet it was a central part of our teaching.

If you listen carefully enough, the patient will tell you the diagnosis.

The most important part of the evaluation is the history.

We were told it over, and over again. And why was it so emphasized? It must have been understood that it's something we could easily do badly.

All I can say in explanation is that Lyme was a "new" disease in 1975.

Physicians are slow to adapt to the new. This innate conservatism has led to many bad examples in the History of Medicine of delay in applying excellent knowledge. Pasteur's discovery of bacteria in the 1850s was not fully accepted until the 1920s.

The arrival of a scientific basis for medical practice and improvements in investigative ability with ease of communication means that things have moved much more quickly over the last eighty years. We adapt better these days.

In the year 2023 I think Lyme is much better understood than it was in 1975. It is a common disease that is getting commoner.

I practice medicine in a cheerful, efficient group practice with colleagues I admire and who are absolutely not dismissive of people complaining of exhaustion, aches and pains with normal blood work. I have a particular interest in such patients; those with the Exhaustion syndrome of whatever cause. So, it came as a shock to read, online, the level of bitterness held against the medical profession that I don't see in my practice. I knew these views were out there I just wasn't aware of their intensity. Here's ten. I am going to keep them anonymous. I offer no comment.

- Doctors don't tell you the truth.
- She says...they dismiss it because they are not educated about it....one doctor told me it was one page at med school…
- ...they have patronizing, condescending attitudes.
- Please miss, why do doctors deny Lymes?
- What about the 17 yr. old boy who died of carditis? He had been ill for a month!
- I was told it couldn't be Lyme because there was no bull's eye.
- You only had four bands; it's got to be five the doctors told me.
- The ex-Nazi Erich Traub injected ticks with *Borrelia burgdorferi* on Plum Island and seagulls flew it off to Lyme, Connecticut. Check the map.
- The CDC are liars.
- Lyme patients suffering from devastating neurological and physical symptoms have desperately been trying to get the CDC to acknowledge that they have a chronic infection that requires further treatment. Yet the CDC continues to ignore the problem.
- If you remain sick after the prescribed length of antibiotic treatment you are a modern medical pariah
- And some people manifest with multiple systemic symptoms that can occur throughout the body, which lead to complex lab results. *Because of this, Lyme disease has been ignored or trivialized by the medical profession for more than a quarter of a century."*

No, I'm sorry I have to interrupt. I can't let this last one stand. *"Because* of multiple symptoms and complex lab results Lyme disease has been ignored or trivialized" ...*What?* I love multiple symptoms with complex lab results! Give me more of them. (Here are ten diseases, off the top of my head, that cause multiple symptoms and have complex lab results, none of which have been ignored or trivialized;

Systemic Lupus Erythematosus
Human Immunodeficiency Virus infection/ AIDS
Tuberculosis
Brucellosis
West Nile Virus
Vasculitis, many kinds
Diabetes
Mono syndrome
Crystal arthropathy
Lymphoma)

Allow me to point out that it was members of this same lying, condescending, pariah-labelling, ignoring, trivializing medical profession that applied the tenets of Science, insisting on the necessity of proving a hypothesis with evidence before accepting it as the truth, that discovered the disease in North America, found the organism that causes it, found a way to epidemiologically monitor it and found a curative therapy with the use of antibiotics (previously discovered by members of this same corrupt medical profession). The CDC has written a 30 -page set of guidelines on how to manage it authored by 34 professors of Medicine from the country's most prestigious universities.

Ignoring? Trivializing? NOT, thank you *very* much.

Or are you suggesting that because of one or two misinformed physicians it is okay to tarnish the entire profession with this calumny? Sir! Or perhaps Madam! You go too far.

At this point I went for a stroll along the beach.

Chapter Ten
"YOU HAVE GOT LYME". ACTUALLY, YOU DON'T.

Having examined the Exhaustion syndrome and seen how many causes of it there are, it is as well to acknowledge that 25 of those hundred patients we discussed earlier do not have an identifiable cause.

Lyme "Literate" doctor (LLD): This patient I just saw, the 35 yr. old man with exhaustion, aches and pains, impaired sleep and brain fog that isn't getting better; therefore, he has Chronic Lyme.

Me: But he was born and raised in Florida, he works in Manhattan, he never had clinical features of Lyme and his tests are negative.

LLD: The tests are notoriously unreliable. There are many false negatives.

Me: There are many causes of this syndrome. Why not follow him up in the office, with supportive care, clinical reassessment including repeating the Lyme and other tests?

LLD: Why not treat him with antibiotics and see if it helps. Just in case. You not wanting to give more antibiotics is demonstrating how little you know about this disease.

Me: I can think of some patients that I might treat with a three-week course of antibiotics, empirically. That is without evidence diagnostic of Lyme disease but a) not this patient, at least not at this time and b) I would not give prolonged courses of intravenous antibiotics as they have serious side effects. Not only are they expensive, they have never been shown to work. Many of these patients recover spontaneously without specific treatments. They are suffering prolonged convalescence from infections like Long Covid.

LLD; Many of them aren't. They have Chronic Lyme.

Chapter Eleven
LYME WARS.

For the last thirty years, conflict between the medical establishment and a selection of doctors, advocacy groups, patients, some puzzled, some angry, and journalists over how to diagnose and treat one simple aspect of this infection, has been so intense it has been dubbed "War". This disagreement is unique in the history of modern Medicine.

What is it about?

15 to 20% of people, treated or not, for Lyme disease develop the Exhaustion syndrome.
Some doctors call this Chronic Lyme and treat with long courses of antibiotics, for six months, a year or even longer.

The Infectious Disease Society of America (IDSA) guidelines thinks that the evidence to support this is dubious and thinks that the dangers of long-term antibiotics outweigh any potential benefit.

The International Lyme and Associated Diseases Society (ILADS) guidelines says that the evidence shows that *Borrelia burgdorferi* bacteria survive short courses of antibiotics in humans and the benefits outweigh the risks.

That's pretty much it. Oh, there are three other disagreements.

1. Tick bite

IDSA recommends two hundred mgs of doxycycline, two tablets,
ILADS recommends 20 days of docycycline 200mgs, two tablets, twice a day

2. Acute Lyme

IDSA recommends 2-4 weeks of doxycycline
ILADS recommends 4-5 weeks.

3. Co-infections

IDSA

There is no evidence for

a) chronic anaplasmosis
b) chronic babesiosis in immunocompetent patients without detectable parasitemia
c) for Babesia duncani in the absence of detectable parasitemia.
d) for tick borne transmission of Bartonella.
e) for simultaneous Lyme disease and Bartonella infection

ILADS states the exact opposite of these five statements.

How does money come into it?

The insurance companies will not pay for courses of antibiotics longer than 28 days because of the IDSA guidelines. The doctors don't make any money out of not giving antibiotics. Their reimbursement is whatever the insurance company pays (with a co-pay from the patient).

ILADS practitioners develop thriving practices from the cost, born by the patient, of antibiotics, special tests not covered by insurance and nutritional supplements.
The patients blame, not the practitioners but the insurance companies for not covering the cost.

I have always tried to be a conscientious objector in this belligerence. It is embarrassing to think that doctors can't get together and reconcile their differences without hostility.

In any case, upcoming improvements in diagnosis and understanding of the mechanism (pathophysiology) of the exhaustion syndrome/chronic Lyme will surely lead to an inevitable amnesty.

Not yet it hasn't.

After a number of skirmishes, the first pitched battle came in 2006. Richard Blumenthal, then Attorney General for the State of Connecticut sued the Infectious Disease Society of America (IDSA) saying that their guidelines for the diagnosis and management of Lyme written by an array of thirty-four scholars; professors of infectious disease, pharmacists and academic entomologists had been falsely rearranged to protect insurance companies from having to pay for prolonged courses of antibiotics. An independent review panel of 8 experts, each agreed to by both sides, unanimously supported the IDSA in 67 of their 68 recommendations and 7-1 in favor of the 68th.

If you thought that such a crushing defeat would have brought hostilities to an end you would be wrong.

Allen Steere, who first described Lyme disease on the North American continent came to think, and wrote in the Journal of the American Medical Association, that most people with Chronic Lyme did not have persistent infection and many of them had never had Lyme in the first place. They were more likely to be suffering from mental illness, or fibromyalgia. "In my opinion" he wrote, "there is no such thing as Chronic Lyme as defined in this way."

Hordes of patients began to stalk him. They showed up at his public engagements showing signs that read "How many more will you kill?" and "Steer clear of Steere."

The first placard would be ironic since prolonged intravenous antibiotic through a venous catheter kills more people than Lyme disease.

In spite of efforts to explain his point of view, the vilification persisted. Public advocates, citizens in number and a coterie of politicians attacked the man who described the disease (on the North American continent) in the first place. In a public senate discussion, he tried to explain why he felt there was over-diagnosis of Chronic Lyme and the crowd began to chant, "He's wrong, he's wrong". He endured death threats. Yes, that's right, people wrote to him and threatened to kill him because he did not think people with the exhaustion syndrome *necessarily* had chronic Lyme disease.

Now, let's stop for a moment and consider the patient. The patient feels sick. The doctor evaluates him/her and finds nothing wrong. Bloodwork and X-rays are normal. The patient may feel dismissed, stigmatized, told that it's all in his/her head, that it is a psychiatric problem.

It is easy to see that he/she will feel restored by another doctor who says "you have Chronic Lyme and I recommend long courses of intravenous antibiotics." It validates them. And if they have a diagnosis, their insurance should respect them. That is the power of the phrase "Chronic Lyme."

The priority, therefore is for establishment physicians to stop delegitimizing the patients' illness, to the extent that they do. Over the last twenty years our approach to these challenging patients has improved. No one, today, in 2023 is denying the reality of the patients' dis-ease.

Yet the war drags on.

In 2017, in Texas, 28 patients with Lyme Disease, sued the IDSA, seven Lyme disease experts who helped write the guidelines, and six national health plans, alleging that the insurance companies paid these experts large consulting fees in a conspiracy to deny treatment and coverage for chronic Lyme disease. Anti-trust and Rico violations were alleged together with common-law fraudulence and negligent misrepresentation against the IDSA.
The allegations of receiving large consulting fees were dropped in the revised lawsuit that ultimately went to trial.

The court dismissed all of the plaintiffs' claims with prejudice. It said, "the plaintiffs did not set forth any affirmative evidence...to support their allegations of a conspiracy to deny the existence of chronic Lyme disease in exchange for payment...they offer merely speculation, conclusory assertions and attorney argument."
Spokesman for the IDSA hailed the rulings as "a victory for patients and for science." What about the other 91 guidelines written by IDSA for all kinds of infectious disease?

I tend to the IDSA side.

The thought of giving long courses of antibiotics, intravenous or oral, makes me shudder. It is against first principles. You are increasing the risk of selecting antibiotic resistant bacteria, you are exposing the patients to the risk of *Clostridium difficile* colitis, line sepsis and blood clots, suppression of the bone marrow and *gallstones*, all of which carries a small but definite mortality. The longer patients are treated, the more likely these side effects are.

So first, do no harm.

One articulate clinical voice for ILADS is Dr Richard Horowitz author of the best-seller "How Can I Get Better? An action plan for treating resistant Lyme and Chronic Disease." Dr Horowitz works in Hyde Park, New York in private practice. He says that he has seen 12,000 patients with Lyme disease.

After reading his book which I recommend I think that what he is talking about is the Exhaustion Syndrome, and not Chronic Lyme, or to think of the phrase "Chronic Lyme" as another synonym.

I particularly like his detailed questionnaire that covers thoroughly the multitudinous causes of the syndrome and is an excellent contribution to how we should be approaching it. He emphasizes the need for an unrushed assessment of the patient, the importance of the history and a personalized approach. I agree with him on all of these points. Needless to say, there are disagreements too. I don't think mycoplasma should be considered a co-infection, protomyxzoa rheumatica is not a pathogen and there is confirmation bias in the assumption that Lyme disease is the basic disease that needs elimination.

A voice for IDSA is Professor Michael Lantos, professor in the department of Family Medicine and Community Health at Duke University. He was chairman of the IDSA guidelines writer's committee.

"Chronic Lyme disease is a poorly defined diagnosis that is usually given to patients with prolonged unexplained symptoms or with alternative medical diagnoses. Data do not support the proposition that chronic, treatment-refractory infection with *Borrelia burgdorferi* is responsible for the many conditions that get labelled as Chronic Lyme disease. Prolonged symptoms after successful treatment of Lyme disease are uncommon, but in rare cases may be severe. Prolonged courses of antibiotics neither prevent nor ameliorate these symptoms and are associated with considerable harm."

The National Institute of Allergy and Infectious Disease, (NIAID) has an active research program into this and other Lyme related questions. It has been impossible to show benefit from the treatments used by the Lyme Literati. The argument is clearly laid out at its website.

Having said that, persistence of *Bb* in tissue, that can grow in culture after standard therapy in non-human primates has been shown. Does persistence of the organism mean it is still capable of causing disease?

That is the great unanswered question, and it is over this question that the War continues.

In 2023 this is where we stand. Only Science can bring the two sides to the table and sign a peace treaty but to date, there is no cease fire in sight. Only Science can end the Lyme Wars.

How will this all seem in a hundred years?
What would Otzi say?

Chapter Twelve
FIVE PATIENTS

1. A 60-year-old University Lecturer
   was encouraged to take early retirement as he was getting forgetful which interfered with his ability to lecture. He saw a neurologist who diagnosed early Alzheimer's. disease. His wife who was born in England took him to London where a second neurologist agreed with this diagnosis. He had the symptoms for over a year and they were gradually worsening.
   He lived in New York City and had a weekend cottage in Hurley west of the Hudson River. He liked nothing better on a Saturday morning than to go for walks through the woods and fields.

   When I spoke to him in the office, in the presence of his wife, he was disorientated and forgetful. He scored badly on the mini mental assessment. The blood test was positive for Lyme. Spinal tap showed eight antibodies to *Bb*, but no active meningitis. CT brain scan showed mild nonspecific abnormalities.
   A diagnosis of neurolyme, also called neuroborreliosis was made and he was treated for four weeks of intravenous Ceftriaxone. Generally, antibiotics prevent worsening of neurological symptoms but there is little improvement. This patient, atypically, showed significant improvement for about a year, and then his cognitive impairment worsened again.

   Comment
   This patient emphasizes the need for early diagnosis. Anyone with impaired cognition living in the Lyme Zone must have the disease excluded before other causes of dementia are accepted.
   When his dementia worsened again at the end of a year, I elected to treat him for a second time with Ceftriaxone for a month. The IDSA guidelines do not recommend this.
   Physicians make clinical decisions based on judgement and experience and as valuable as the IDSA document is, it is as its name suggests, a Guideline. And in the preamble this fact is emphasized
   This time his symptoms did not improve and he stayed in a state of mild to moderate dementia. Little change was noted over a three year follow up.

2. A 75-year-old retired schoolteacher.
   Main complaint: deafness in his left ear getting worse over the last seven years.

History; "it's due to Lyme disease, doctor. I've been under treatment with a famous Lyme doctor who has been treating me for the last nine months with intravenous antibiotics through this line." He showed me the catheter placed in a vein in his arm.

Was that his only treatment?

"No, I get a package of vitamins and other drugs delivered once a week to my house"

Why did he say your deafness was due to Lyme disease?

"Well, he sent off some blood to a lab in North Dakota, because the routine ones were all negative."

Did you see an ENT doctor?

"No, there was no need he told me. Don't get me wrong, I like Dr X, I just can't afford him anymore. The antibiotics are a thousand a month. The vitamins cost $350. I just want to continue the antibiotics on my retirement insurance benefit. That's why I came to see you. You take insurance. This has made a big dent on my retirement savings"

Have you noticed any improvement in your hearing?

"No, he said it would be slow and might take a year or so."

How do you feel generally in yourself?

"No, I'm fine. I exercise regularly, I play golf twice a week."

Comment:

Lyme disease can cause hearing loss in one or both ears. In the acute or early disseminated phase of the disease it usually causes sudden onset of deafness. Progressive deafness in late disseminated Lyme disease is usually bilateral. Usually, but not always. It may also be associated with tinnitus, (ringing in the ears) and vertigo.

This patient had no other features of Lyme. His cognitive testing was normal /excellent. Standard antibody testing for Lyme was negative.

Hearing loss in the elderly is extremely common. A staggering 35% of people over the age of 50 are affected. The commonest cause is presbyacusis or decline in efficient neurological function with age. Often there is a combination of causes.

Antibiotics for deafness due to Lyme disease may have some benefit. What we know is based on anecdotes but in most cases the symptom does not improve and there is no indication to give long courses of drugs (i.e., greater than two to four weeks), which is potentially dangerous in itself, particularly if there is no improvement over that time.

I referred this patient to an ENT doctor who evaluated him carefully. I would like to report that he had an acoustic neuroma and this was surgically removed with return of his hearing, but mild loss was found in the other ear and the diagnosis of presbyacusis was made. I recommended stopping the antibiotics and removing the intravenous line. He was a little reluctant to accept this, so I arranged for a second opinion with another ENT doctor in town with a lot of experience with Lyme disease and deafness. He agreed with the first ENT doctor. A year later I was still seeing him in follow up and although his general health was excellent, there was little change in his earing loss.

Comment; Just because you can't say it isn't Lyme, doesn't mean it is.

3. A 42-year-old real estate agent said to me

    "I have Lyme again, could you give me some doxycycline?"

    What are your symptoms

    "Oh, I just feel generally run down"

    Have you been bitten by a tick?

    "Years ago. Look I felt just the same way as I do now about eighteen months ago when I had Lyme and I took some doxycycline then and got immediate improvement, so that's what I would like now."

    What made you think it was Lyme back then? Did you have 'flu? a red spot?

    He grinned sheepishly.

    "I knew it was Lyme because my cousin had the same thing and he was told it was Lyme. I researched it on line. So, there was no need to see a doctor. My wife had some doxycycline left over that she never took. And that's how I got it. Look, I know you're a busy man and all I really want is a prescription, so...

    "People usually say we are too much in a hurry, that we don't spend enough time with our patients."

    I asked him a few more questions. He did have some aches and pains in his joints he told me but no fever and no previous illness "except the Lyme"

    Examination was within normal limits. I got him to agree to have some blood tests. It wasn't easy. His blood tests came back negative for Lyme disease, he had mild anemia and a positive ANA test which is often associated with auto-immune disease.

    Comment

    Dr Google is not a bad thing, necessarily, when carefully consulted. Patients can't have too much information about their diseases, but there is such a wide variety of unsubstantiated opinion online that objectivity and truth can be drowned out.

    You can say for certain that this patient did not have Lyme disease the first time when he diagnosed himself with it. His antibody test, a year after an episode of acute Lyme would be positive. His was negative.

    His positive ANA test might be harmless or it might be a sign of vasculitic disease. This would require more detailed assessment including the opinion of a Rheumatologist. He would not agree to my recommendations; "I know I have Lyme".

    A delusion is a false belief that is held, despite evidence to the contrary, that cannot be influenced by logic.

    It is of interest to note that doxycycline has anti-inflammatory properties as well as antibiotic action and this may have helped his joint pains. I prescribed a fourteen-day course of doxycyline, on the grounds that he might have acute Lyme this time and to see how it made him feel. I made an appointment for him to see a rheumatologist He took the prescription but did not follow up.

4. Patient A and Patient B were both 65-year-old newly retired women. Both were healthy without chronic disease. They presented with similar illnesses. Both developed weakness of the right side of the face, a general sense of malaise and a low-grade fever. Their blood tests were positive

for Lyme antibodies and a spinal tap was normal in both patients. They were treated with oral doxycycline for three weeks with initial improvement and recovery of the facial paralyses.

They each returned to the office a month later complaining of general weakness. Six months later, the symptoms persisted.

Patient A felt tired all the time, her sleep was disturbed. She had aches and pains in her muscle and joints and felt generally apathetic. Both suffered "brain-fog".

Patient B had a dull aching in her back and headaches to which she was not usually prone. Both felt tired all the time Examination, of both, was normal. Their previous facial weakness was undetectable. Routine blood work was in the normal range.

History taking is always important, but it is particularly so when interacting with patients complaining of the Exhaustion syndrome. The concept of using a detailed questionnaire is excellent and I use one based on the General System Questionnaire 30 of Dr Daniel Cameron, but note that Dr Horowitz also has a questionnaire that is available online.

Both patients showed high scores. One value of the questionnaire is that it can be used repeatedly over time to measure improvement or deterioration.

The diagnosis in each case was Post Treatment Lyme Disease Syndrome.

I recommended fresh air and vitamins. Regular exercise of moderate degree avoiding overexertion, the avoidance of stress to the extent it was possible. Patient B took up Yoga. Above all I offered strong reassurance to both and predicted slow but definite recovery.

They asked pertinent questions;

What is the cause of PTLDS?

To date that is unknown. Current research into Long Covid may shed light on the common phenomenon of prolonged convalescence after an acute infection.

The leading hypotheses are a) a delayed response of the immune system, b) the persistence of infection, c) some unrelated factor. Think of it as Long Lyme. Why some people get it while the majority do not is poorly understood.

Would more antibiotics help?

Probably not. The NIH has performed studies that show no benefit from long courses of antibiotics. Moreover, they have potentially serious side effects.

Patient B accepted this. She continued to suffer from PTLDS for a further 12 months with gradual improvement after six. She returned to her normal state of good health Patient A sought a second opinion with "alternative" doctors. She had a prolonged course of antibiotics for six months which she tolerated except for a little diarrhea, had hyperbaric oxygen treatment, chelation and heavy metal therapy, immunoglobulin infusions with minimal nausea, headache and rash, and spiritual counselling. She continued to suffer from PTLDS for a further 12 months with gradual improvement after six. This improvement was attributed to the treatments she had taken. She returned to her normal state of good health

COMMENT. No comment.

5. A 52-yr-old man who has been a farmer in the Mid-Hudson Valley all his working life. He is outdoors for ten hours a day and has been bitten many times by ticks.

He has never knowingly had Lyme disease or any other febrile illness except for flu some twenty years ago.

For the last two months, he has complained of increasing tiredness. This is not like him. He sleeps long hours but wakes up exhausted and often has to nap in the afternoons.

"I can't think straight" he says, "the simplest task seems impossible, I have lost interest in doing anything. I have these mysterious aches and pains, there is something wrong Doc, this isn't me."

He fills out the questionnaire.

We discuss his kids. One of them had Lyme, was treated and he is better now. The patient himself is wearing a Yankee cap. He used to be a fan but now he can't be bothered to turn on the TV.

He is carefully examined. No abnormality is detected. A thorough workup with blood test and X-rays is performed. The results are all in the normal range. The Lyme antibody test with western blot is normal.

SHOULD THIS MAN BE TREATED FOR LYME DISEASE?

COMMENT

Since the treatment would be four weeks of doxycycline 100mgs bid, a low risk regimen, you might ask, what would be the downside?

Well, antibiotics have side effects, and should be used with care. Although this man lives in a high-risk environment, his antibody test is negative. He has been ill for three months so you could have predicted positive serology.

A spinal tap is performed.

His cerebrospinal fluid is entirely normal with no Bb antibodies detected.

Since it is important to exclude named organic disease, meticulous revaluation of the clinical features and appropriate bloodwork, possibly with a second opinion from a fellow Infectious Diseases specialist should be the next step, with close, say weekly follow up.

It would not be unreasonable for a clinician who could find no other cause for this man's symptoms to give two to four weeks of doxycycline.

Part Four
THE ESSENTIALS

What follows are practical matters that may be read as reference.

Chapter Thirteen
BORRELIA BURGDORFERI IS A SPIROCHETE.

Bacteria have been on earth for 3.5 billion years.
One family (order) of bacteria is called Spirochetae.

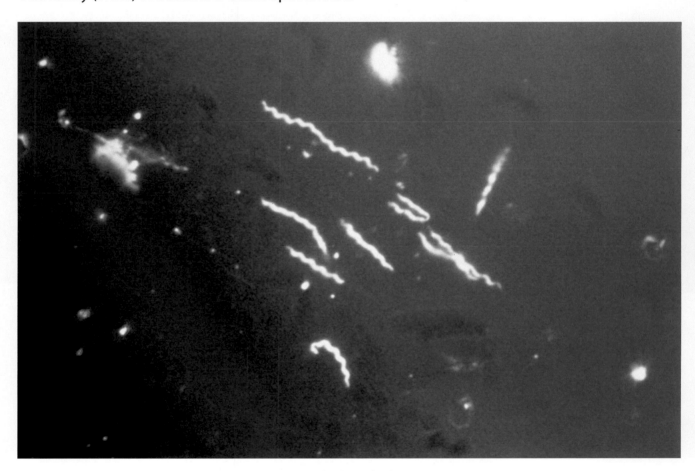

Borrelia burgdorferi.
Source: CDC

These unique corkscrew shaped microorganisms live without oxygen which suggests they evolved before the Great Oxidation Event 2.5 billion years ago.

Spirochetes can be seen in the stomachs of ticks trapped in amber from what is now the Dominican Republic between 15 to 20 million years ago.

Spirocheteness is helical.

The two most frequent human spirochetal diseases in the world are:

Syphilis	*Treponema pallidum.*
Lyme Disease	*Borrelia burgdorferi* sensu lato (broad sense)

<u>They have in common</u>.
The portal of entry is skin or mucus membranes
They disseminate widely in the body
They evade immunity
They enter the central nervous system early in the disease.
They have stages with intervening latent phases
Untreated infections may last from months to decades.
They both cause a treatable form of dementia.
<u>But:</u>
They are different in biochemistry and structure and are categorized in different families. Lyme disease cannot be acquired from sex and Syphilis is not transmitted by a tick.

There are a number of closely related Borrrelia species that come under the heading of Borrelia burgdorferi *sensu lato,* meaning, *in a broad sense.*
In North America; *Borrelia mayonii,* so far only found in the upper Mid-West. Unlike *Bb* it is more likely to cause nausea and vomiting and widespread rash.
Borrelia miyamotoi, Acute febrile illness. Rash unusual. First discovered in Japan, but found around the world.
Europe/Asia; *Borrelia afzelii,* Lyme syndrome. More likely to cause unusual skin diseases such as Morphoea and Acrodermatitis chronica atrophicans.
Borrelia garinii. Lyme syndrome; Particularly likely to cause nerve root pain often referred to as as Bannwarth's syndrome.
   Borrelia spielmanii and *Borrelia bavariensis* are also found in Europe.

Other spirochetal diseases:
Leptospirosis
Yaws and Pinta
Rat-bite fever
Relapsing fever
Intestinal spirochetosis, a diarrheal illness
Gingivitis

A number of infections in livestock and wild animals.

Most spirochete families do not cause disease. We all have spirochetes that live in our mouths and intestines as harmless commensals.

Chapter Fourteen
THE HISTORY OF BORRELIA BURGDORFERI (Bb)

Sequencing the DNA of the genomes of hundreds of Spirochetes and arranging them into an evolutionary tree shows that *Bb* was present in Europe before it reached North America, probably carried by birds, before the last Ice Age.

It got there at least 60,000 years ago, long before the first humans crossed the Bering Strait 24,000 years ago. It was first present in the northeast and spread south and west across the landmass.

Otzi the iceman, the first human known to have Lyme disease proven by DNA studies, died 3,300 years ago in what is now the Austrian Tyrol.

From Otzi's time to Alfred Buchwald's first published clinical description of Lyme, the rash *acrodermatitis chronica atrophicans* in 1883 in Breslau, Germany, now Wroclaw, Poland the number of people who suffered from *Bb* infection must have run into the hundreds of thousands. Yet it has left a very small mark on human history. But then, *H sapiens* had not heard of and had no understanding of bacteria. "Lyme" was not acutely lethal, and its diverse chronic features could not be explained as one entity.

Until recent times, references to Lyme disease in history are unprovable. In the 18th century there was an outbreak of arthritis on the Hebridean island of Jura (which means Deer in Norse). Many ticks were noted by travelers. To this day Lyme is commoner in Scotland than any other part of the UK.

In America there are descriptions of Lyme like symptoms and disease in the 17th and 18th centuries amongst the American colonialists with much reference being made by travellers to the large numbers of ticks interfering with their explorations.

Dr MM Drymon has written two books about how plagues, particularly Lyme disease, affect culture and makes a convincing case that the *stigmata diabolito*, the mark the devil leaves on witches referred to in the Salem witch trials of 1690 in Massachussetts, were ECM rashes. She also considers that the mental state of the "witches" might have been a consequence of Lyme infection.

DNA analyses from museum specimens of stuffed animals reveal the bacteria were present on Cape Cod in the 1890s, and Long Island in the 1940s before clinical recognition of the disease in America.

Lyme disease in Europe followed three phases; first the descriptive. Following Buchwald's work, Arfid Afzelius, a Swedish dermatologist, presented cases of Erythema Chronicum Migrans in 1909, publishing his findings 12 years later. He attributed it to the bite of a tick and was recognized for his discovery by having a specie of Borrelia named after him, *Borrelia Afzelii*, the commonest cause of Lyme disease in Europe.

In 1941 in Germany, Alfred Bannwarth described radiculitis that is to say inflammation of the nerve as it leaves the spinal cord leading to pain. Sciatica is a common example of this syndrome. Bannwarth practiced through the war, enlisted in 1945, was immediately captured by the Allies and spent the next year as a prisoner of war. He showed that radiculopathy could have an infectious cause and European physicians went on to show that this infection responded to Penicillin. This was phase two, the therapeutic.

In 1975, Alan Steere, from Yale University, described this infectious disease in Lyme Connecticut while investigating an outbreak of arthritis in children. Like Bannwarth he had studied music before taking up Medicine. He named the disease after the town in which it was described. This was the first description of Lyme disease on the North American continent.

The bacteria that cause Lyme disease was discovered by the Swiss born Dr Willy Burgdorfer, working out of the Rocky Mountain laboratories in Montana in 1981.

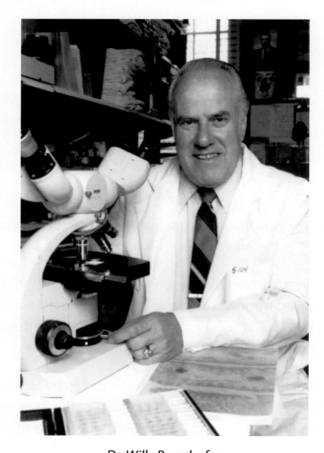

Dr. Willy Burgdorfer.

Back in Europe, the name Lyme disease was widely accepted and is now commonly used leading to stage three; outlining the epidemiology, looking at the difference between European and American disease, categorizing its nature and establishing its place as a bacterial infection.

Lyme disease is a now a global pandemic augmented by environmental factors; in particular ticks are expanding their habitat with global warming.

In the northeast of the United States there has been a huge increase in the deer herd; this together with a long history of deforestation and reforestation with extensive suburbanization explains the high prevalence of the disease there.

Chapter Fifteen
TICKS

They are small spider like creatures that feed on the blood of birds and mammals such as humans. Most are harmless to man.

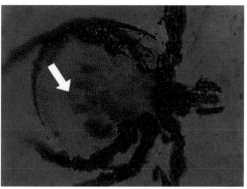

Tick in amber. The arrow indicates a spirochete in its intestine.
Courtesy of Prof. George Poinar Jr.

Amber is fossilized tree resin. Insects, cuckoo wasps, soldier flies, beetles and ticks have been trapped in amber and preserved from 99 million years ago when dinosaurs roamed the planet. The Dominican Republic, as it is known today, has copious amber on its northern coastline, which is where this sample was found.

This picture shows a larval tick of the same Ixodes species as transmits Lyme today. You will see spirochete like cells, closely resembling Borrelia in the lumen of the insect's alimentary tract. This tick is estimated to be 15 million years old by radiocarbon dating the rocks that surround it.

We (*Homo sapiens*) appeared on the planet 300,000 years ago.

The oldest known tick fossils are around a hundred million years old. Today, they live in every climate on every continent. There are 850 species in the world, but "only" 90 in the United States, where there are two families; the hard ticks (Ixodids) and the soft ticks (Argasids). They are active year-round.

They infect dogs. Dogs and other animals bring them into the house.

They do not fly. They are found on fallen leaves, grasses and bushes. They attach to animals brushing past them. This is called questing. What sort of technique of replication is this you may ask? How's that going to work?

They have been around for 99 million years.

They grasp the skin, cut into it inserting its feeding tube secreting a cement like substance that keeps them attached with tenacity. They fall off when full.

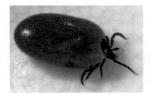

A bloated tick.
Source: CDC/Dr. Gary Alpert

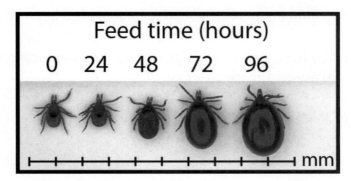

The life cycle of Ixodes, the deer tick.
Source: CDC.

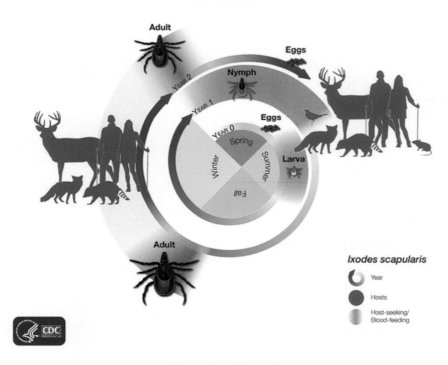

Life cycle of the tick.
Source: CDC

The life cycle of the tick Is complicated and lasts two years. There are four stages, eggs, six-legged larva eight legged nymphs and eight-legged adult.

Larvae hatch nymphs and they both may eat *Borrelia burgdorferi* whilst sucking blood. The white footed mouse, birds, humans and other animals are the hosts. Then nymphs and adults transmit it to humans and other animals. Most Lyme is transmitted to man by nymphs from May through July.

They do not transmit microbes until they have fed for 24 hours. There are exceptions to this general rule.

List of diseases transmitted by ticks, in the USA and organisms capable of co-infecting with Lyme.

Babesia microti is the commonest specie to cause disease in the USA, whereas in Europe is it *Babesia divergens*. In 1991 a new Babesia organism, transmitted by ticks was identified in Washington state. Its name is *Babesia duncani-WA 1*. It looks the same as *microti* but it genetically different. It is found across the United States but has been most reported from the Pacific Northwest and Canada.

The rarest form to cause human disease, *Babesia venatorum,* has been described in China, Europe and the United States.

All four are transmitted by ticks, infect a wide group of animals including *Homo sapiens* and cause similar disease ranging from asymptomatic to lethal.

Here is the formal list of all microbes transmitted by ticks known to date.

A: In the United States

Anaplasmosis
Babesiosis
Borrelia burgdorferi
Borrelia mayonii
Borrelia myamotoi
Bourbon virus
Colorado Tick Fever
Ehrlichiosis
Heartland virus
Lyme disease
Powassan
Rickettsia parkeri
Rocky Mountain Spotted Fever
STARI, Southern tick-associated rash illness
Tick borne relapsing fever
Tularemia
364D rickettsiosis
These can also be acquired internationally.

B: Outside of the United States.

Borrelia afzeli
Borrelia bavariensis
Borrelia garinii.
Borrelia spielmanii

Crimea-Congo hemorrhagic fever (virus)
Rickettsiae africae, african spotted fever
Fièvre boutonneuse, rickettsial, Mediterranean littoral.
Brazilian spotted fever
Scrub typhus
Kyasanur forest disease, Southern India (virus). a
Tickborne encephalitis (virus)
Omsk hemrrorrhagic fever (virus)

<u>What to do if you are bitten by a tick?</u>

In the Lyme Zone, everyone is at risk, but you are particularly so if you hike, hunt, garden, play golf or are outside in the tall grass for any reason.
You should therefore take precautions. Wear long sleeves and tuck your pants into your socks.
N, N-Diethyl-meta-toluamide (DEET) is an excellent and safe insecticide to put on your exposed skin surface. You can also use picaridin, oil of lemon eucalyptus, or permethrin.
Note that wood ticks are quite large whereas *Ixodes scapularis* (IS) the transporters of disease are tiny. If you are bitten by any tick, you are at risk for also being bitten by the Lyme tick so I recommend a shower if you have been at high-risk activity with rough toweling to pull off those *ixodes* that might be found in the hairline or on the back or behind the knee or other such places that might miss a tick inspection.

If the tick is attached remove it. This may prove more difficult than you think, they are tenacious little insects. Don't try to burn them off, it doesn't work and it may hurt.
Use a clean fine tipped tweezer and push it between the tick body and the skin.

Best practice is to take the tick to the doctor and if it is diagnosed as *ixodes* that is valuable information but if it isn't you are still at risk for having been bitten by IS. If you are bitten by one tick species you are at risk of having been bitten by another.

You may elect to take two tablets of doxycycline 100mgs each and most providers would prescribe this. It has some prophylactic value but is by no means absolutely protective. Some practitioners would give a two-week course of treatment for a tick bite.

Such recommendations regarding clothing and insecticides are frequently not followed, particularly by children. In this case after a day at risk in the fields, the shower followed by rough toweling is the best preventative step.

Chapter Sixteen
THE LYME ZONE

The map below shows where Lyme disease has been documented.

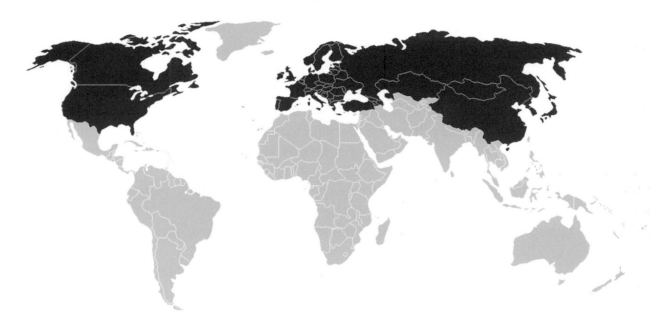

Geographical distribution of Lyme disease cases.
Source: Wikimedia Commons

One survey writes that 14% of humans world-wide have been infected with Lyme disease. That's 1 in 7. It is particularly well documented in the temperate zone of the Northern Hemisphere.

What about the Southern Hemisphere?

Australia

People can acquire Lyme disease elsewhere in the world and bring it back to Australia but the scientific community there does not accept the diagnosis of locally acquired infection. *Borrelia burgdorferi* has not been found in any Australian ticks or any other Australian insect vector that passes the disease to humans.

In spite of this there is an active practice for people with fatigue who are convinced that they have Lyme disease and pay many thousands of dollars for unproven long term therapies including antibiotics.

Local practitioners recognize a group of patients with fatigue, disordered thinking, disordered sleep, joint pains, muscle pains attributed by some to tick bites. It is called Debilitating Symptom Complexes attributed to Ticks. (DSCATT). We can add this to the list of synonyms for the Exhaustion syndrome.

The Australian equivalent of ILADS, the Lyme Disease Association of Australia, LDAA disagrees and says that there is *Borrelia Burgdorferi* infection in Australia.

India

In 2018, a case report of undoubted Lyme disease was published in Tropical Doctor 48(4) 004947551878955 by Tewatia P, et al.
This has been followed by further series of case reports that establish that Lyme disease undoubtedly exists in India, but so far has only been found in the North.

Pakistan

Tick borne illnesses such as Anaplasmosis and Babesiosis exist in Pakistan but to date there are no reports of Lyme disease.

Africa

Africa is a vast continent made up of 54 countries. It is impossible therefore to exclude the existence of Lyme disease there. but to date there are no reports of such.

Brazil

A disease similar to Lyme called the Baggio-Yoshinari syndrome, first described in 1992, is a rare disease found in several areas of the country that is transmitted by ticks. It is caused by a *Borrelia* bacteria that responds well to antibiotics. A similar possibility exists in Argentina, yet if the disease does exist there it does not appear to be well recognized. Llamas and Alpacas may carry certain human pathogens (Yersinia) but not Borrelia.

Chapter Seventeen
DIAGNOSTIC TESTS

Current antibody tests for Lyme disease are useful but imperfect.

That is true for the majority of tests in use. False positives and false negatives are part of everyday clinical life and not just Lyme disease. Better tests are awaited, but the ones we have are pretty good particularly when you understand their limitations. They are to be interpreted in the light of the symptoms and signs of the patient's illness. What is the likelihood he or she has been exposed to black legged ticks? Is there another illness that might cause these symptoms and signs? Acute Lyme with an EM rash is treated without any testing, as are some patients without an EM rash. It would be thorough to follow up testing at six to eight weeks but this requires the cooperation of the patient.

The standard tests that detect antibodies are:

Indirect Fluorescent Antibodies (IFA)
Enzyme linked immunosorbent assay (ELISA)

When one of these is performed, if negative, no further testing is needed, if positive or equivocal, a second confirmatory test, called a Western Blot, is performed. This is the two-tier system. Usually, the two tests are ordered at the same time.

We have seen that in acute Lyme the test(s) are usually negative. When antibodies appear they persist for years, long after the infection is gone. They do tend to diminish over time and when they do, this can be taken as objective evidence of cure. Before accepting this, be careful to exclude neurological disease. In neurological disease, the serum test may be negative but the CSF test will be positive 87% of the time.

In Lyme arthritis the tests are close to 100% specific and sensitive.

False positives are occasional, less than ten percent of the time. It means that first, there is some other cause for the patient's symptoms, and second, the patient may have received a course of antibiotics they did not need.

False negatives are much more serious. If Lyme is untreated, severe late complications may occur, so clinicians are more likely to overtreat than undertreat. Treating for two to four weeks of oral doxycycline is not the same as giving patients months or even years of antibiotics through an intravenous catheter.

There are a range of other tests less commonly used, either because they take too long, require more technological ability than is conveniently available, or because they are not going to change treatment.

A Polymerase Chain Reaction (PCR), which is a means of amplifying specifically and uniquely Bb DNA. It is most helpful when looking at the CSF for central nervous system Lyme but even there has a low sensitivity.

Blood culture has a low yield and is rarely performed.

There are many other tests that have not, so far, been validated by the US Food and Drug Administration.

These include:

FISH test; (Fluorescent in situ hybridization) - detects pathogen's RNA
Capture assays for antigens in the urine
Lymphocyte transformation
CD57 assays
Reverse western blots
Culture enhanced PCR.

Chapter Eighteen
TREATMENT OF LYME DISEASE: ANTIBIOTICS

Penicillin, discovered in 1928, kills bacteria before they kill you. Many antibiotics, ironically, are synthesized in Nature by bacteria or fungi. These powerful compounds evolved to kill other microbes in a battle for survival.

Ancient societies knew this. Mayans used "Cuxum", a folk medicine made from molds and fungi to treat wounds. In the Middle Ages, European peasants used moldy bread for the same purpose. But our oldest knowledge of the historical use of antibiotics is the finding of tetracycline in the bones of Nubians (Sudanese) who died two thousand years ago. They put it in the beer. The ability of growing bacteria to suppress the growth of other bacteria was observed by a number of scientists before Fleming discovered penicillin.

Louis Pasteur himself spoke of *antagonisme microbien* "microbial antagonism" in 1877.

When, in 1982, Dr Wilhelm Burgdorfer showed that *Borrelia burgdorfer,* was the cause of Lyme disease, it was a surprise. Many "had an intuition" the agent would be a virus.

Give antibiotics! was the next thought and an effective therapy it turned out to be.

In 1967 Doxycycline was approved for use in the USA by the Food and Drug Administration. It works by binding to the bacteria's double stranded DNA, making protein synthesis impossible in the microbe, leading to its death. It is standard treatment for acute Lyme, with a 90% cure rate.

It kills a broad spectrum of bacteria with low toxicity. It should not be used in pregnant or lactating women, when Amoxicillin or Cefuroxime is an alternative.

The commonest side effect of doxycycline is nausea, vomiting and diarrhea, which may be severe enough to warrant changing antibiotics in 5% of people who take it.

Absorption is impaired by aluminum, calcium, iron or magnesium. These elements are found in anti-indigestion medicines which should not be taken when using doxycycline.

Since it may cause gastrointestinal symptoms, it is important to advise patients to avoid antacids and similar drugs.

Doxycycline is notorious for causing excessive sunburn when the skin is exposed to ultraviolet light. The mechanism of this photosensitivity is unknown. The patient must be told of this so that he or she can avoid sunlight or dress appropriately, while taking the drug.

Alcohol may inhibit the action of doxycycline and, conversely, it may make intoxication easier to achieve. The efficacy of oral contraception may be impaired and the disease SLE may be exacerbated.

Doxycycline should be used with caution in patients with underlying kidney disease as it may, rarely, cause renal failure. Occasionally it may cause inflammation in the liver - hepatitis.

For central nervous system infections or severe acute Lyme, Ceftriaxone, administered intravenously is the antibiotic of choice. It crosses the blood-brain barrier. Studies in Europe show that doxycycline taken by mouth can cure even these more severe infections. Ceftriaxone is excreted through the liver and may cause hepatitis. Prolonged use may lead to the formation of gallstones. Allergy to these antibiotics occurs in about 1% of the population and patients should be routinely questioned about having a known allergy. A patient who cannot take doxycycline, e.g., because of pregnancy, and who has a severe penicillin allergy should be treated with Azithromycin.

Jarisch-Herxheimer (JHR) reaction after treatment for Lyme

In the late 19th century, the Austrian dermatologist Jarisch noted that some patients being treated with mercury for syphilis developed a feverish reaction within 24hrs of starting treatment. Shaking chills, worsening of rashes and a large number of less frequent clinical features would sicken the patient. The symptoms rarely lasted longer than five hours. Two years later, this was confirmed by the German physician Herxheimer.

This discovery was forty years before penicillin was first used to treat the disease, which then led to a similar JHR reaction in a variable percentage of treated patient from 7-30%, depending on the survey. It is usually transient and like the mercury induced reaction, rarely lasts longer than five hours.

JHR has been described in other spirochetal infections including Lyme Disease and there are a number of case reports showing it is a definite phenomenon. The incidence is lower in Lyme than in Syphilis, and from my own experience it is rare. It is popularly known as "herxing".

It has also been attributed to treatment for tick borne infections other than Lyme.

Vaccine

In principle, you would have thought that a vaccine for Lyme disease would be very popular and in wide demand. When Lymerix, found to be safe and effective in trials, came on the market in 1998 it was not successful because it was widely thought to cause severe side effects, in conflict with the trial data. In 2002, citing poor sales, SmithKline Beecham voluntarily withdrew the vaccine.

A related dog vaccine has been very successful.

<u>Herbal treatment for Lyme disease</u>

In the Medical Pharmacy many drugs are first discovered in plants. Morphine from the poppy; digitalis from the foxglove; vincristine, a chemotherapy agent, from the periwinkle. There are many more. It might be given as evidence that if a treatment works it immediately becomes orthodox.

In the therapy of acute and disseminated Lyme disease there is no definitive herbal cure to date but the use of herbs and essential oils may improve the patient's general well-being.

A number of plants.......

Cryptolepis sanguinolenta-Ghanaian quinine
Juglans nigra-Black walnut
Polygonum cuspidatum - Japanese knotweed
Artemisia annua-Sweet wormwood
Uncaria Tomentosa-Cat's claw
Cistus incanus-Rockrose
Scutellaria baicalensis - Chinese skullcap

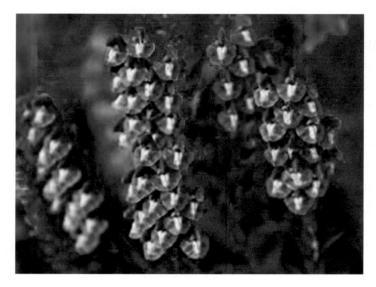

Scutellaria baicalensis - Chinese Scullcap

... have been shown in mice to inhibit or kill "persister" bacteria that are resistant to antibiotics. It is to be hoped that when follow up studies demonstrate similar effects in humans it will cure them of PTLDS.

Chapter Nineteen
TREATMENT OF POST TREATMENT LYME DISEASE SYNDROME (PTLDS).

To recapitulate, PTLDS is one cause of the Exhaustion Syndrome. It occurs in patients who have been diagnosed and treated for Lyme disease, who continue to feel unwell with fatigue, muscle and joint pains, poor sleep, malaise and brain fog. Once objective evidence of organic disease has been excluded by means of history exam and tests, and is not found, how do we treat this illness?

The doctor patient relationship is a crucial part of the management of all illness. You could write a book about it. In fact, quite a few people have. I recommend, *What Patients Say, What Doctors Hear* by Danielle Offri MD. (see bibliography.)

This is nowhere of more importance than in the management of PTLDS. We have seen how disbelieving, supercilious, non-listening doctors have in the past driven patients into the arms of alternative practitioners, charlatans and quacks. If the patient has a good chance of recovery over six months to two years, an empathetic commitment from his or her physician is obviously needed.

So, only connect.

How do you do that?

Listen to the patient. Show empathy. Answer questions directly with clarity.

Reassurance is a powerful tool.

Papers have been published advocating the use of the antibiotics, Dapsone or Disulfiram for the treatment of PTLDS. The underlying hypothesis is that in vitro studies with experimental animals, including chimpanzees have shown persister strains of bacteria, including biofilm forms that live on after treatment with antibiotics. The suggestion is that these organisms cause PTLDS, an entirely reasonable hypothesis. In vitro studies show that although these "persisters" are resistant to standard antibiotics they are destroyed by Dapsone or Disulfiram.

Blinded randomized placebo-controlled trials are awaited. The drugs are not without toxicity. They may be considered for use in severe cases that are not responding to the supportive measures recommended below.

There is a selection of non-antibiotic medicines that can be used with benefit. The clinician will select those he thinks appropriate to the needs and responses of a given patient.

Fish oil.

Naltrexone, good for aches and pains

Gabapentin and Pregabalin.

Dual serotonin and norepinephrine reuptake inhibitors, SNRIs - Cymbalta

Tricyclic antidepressants - Flexeril

SSRTIs - Prozac

There is a definite element of trial and error with these drugs. My experience is that a small number of patients improve miraculously, whereas most get a variable benefit and a very few get none.

For selected patients group therapy is helpful.

Cognitive behavioral therapy. The patient meets with a therapist once a week or once every two weeks to talk over their symptoms and how best they may be dealt with.

Exercise is well known to increase well-being. Low impact aerobic exercise, such as walking or swimming would be recommended.

This can be combined with ancient health programs such as Chinese Qi gong and Tai chi, or Indian Yoga. There are scientific studies that have looked at these activities. Most of them look at 60-minute sessions two to three times a week for 6 to 12 weeks.

Under these conditions, all three significantly improved symptoms of fatigue and sleep quality.

They also have positive effects on anxiety, stress, depression and overall quality of life.

Some find Meditation helpful.

Massage

There is a large body of scientific studies testifying to the use of massage in this condition.

Acupuncture is safe and many people find benefit from it. It is not supported by strong scientific evidence. The FDA approves acupuncture needles as a Class II medical device and requires the needles to be sterile, single use and only to be used appropriately by licensed practitioners.

Chapter Twenty
UNPROVEN TREATMENTS FOR LYME

There are at least thirty treatments used by quacks that don't work.

(Quack - a fraudulent or ignorant pretender to medical skill.)

Adverts rely on testimonials and anecdotes with a veneer of scientific terminology.

This should arouse suspicion that might increase when the cost, often substantial, of the "therapy" is revealed. Or conversely it may lead to the *argumentum ad crumenam* fallacy, that it is better because it is more expensive. It is in the interest of the purveyors of these treatments to devalue science, to talk about the complexity of Lyme and how difficult it is to manage, and to attack the values and attitudes of orthodox practitioners.

Patients are attracted to alternative practitioners when they have chronically unexplained symptoms, false positive, or coincidentally positive tests and occasional psychiatric co-morbidities. They often feel rejected or stigmatized by the Medical Profession.

Patients with the Exhaustion Syndrome often labelled Chronic Lyme may particularly be attracted to these doctors.

There will always be people convinced that they have Lyme disease when they don't, and no amount of debate, argument or scientific proof will change their minds.

There have always been quacks, and there always will be. The era of the internet has increased their number and influence.

The following treatments may be actively harmful,

Bismuth therapy in the drug Bismacine marketed to cure Lyme has caused at least two deaths and is explicitly warned against by the U. S. Food and Drug Administration.

Hyperbaric oxygen

Rectal or vaginal insufflation with gaseous ozone

Ultraviolet light by reinfusion

Removal of dental amalgam.

Apheresis or extracorporeal filtration and replacement of your blood.

Stem cell transplants

<u>The following treatments are Ineffective against Lyme disease</u>

Rife
Use of ozone,
Hydrogen peroxide
Salt/Vitamin C
Glutathione
Moxibustion… burning mugwort root.
Earthworm derived lumbrokinase, soybean derived nattokinase
Chelation and heavy metal therapy
Ingestion of one's own urine
Enemas
Olmesartan
Bleach
Ivermectin
Bee venom
Immune globulin
Cholestyramine-atovaquone

CONCLUSION

"I love everything in the world. Except for ticks." – Dalai Lama.

Life before public hygiene, vaccination and antibiotics was perilous for *Homo sapiens*. In countries where these defenses are missing, it still is.

In 2019, 13.7 million people died of infectious disease.

The three most lethal infections are Tuberculosis - 1.5 million per year; Malaria - 700,000 per year, 75% of which are children under 5, which equals one child per minute; Aids - 600,000 per year.

Developed countries with defenses in place remain vulnerable to pandemics, and our deforestation activities, wildlife trade, population growth, climate change and ease of transport for the pathogens, undermine what has been achieved.

While Lyme disease is not as lethal as these other infections there is an increase in incidence year after year across the northern hemisphere. One in 7 people worldwide are currently infected or have previously had the disease. Central Europe, Western Europe and Eastern Asia have the highest incidences. In the USA there are about 300,000 new infections per year and rising.

Globally, 11 deaths have been reported between 1985 and 2019. As always, we must factor in significant under reporting to this number. If we multiply it by ten thousand it is still less than 0.001% of all Lyme cases that die in the world.

When the diagnosis is made, treatment with antibiotics is highly effective. With society's partial mastery of lethal infectious diseases comes better health and longer life. The non-lethal Exhaustion syndrome, known for at least two thousand years, becomes more prominent in such a society. Approximately 15% of people diagnosed and treated for acute Lyme develop PTLDS.

PTLDS is indistinguishable from

Fibromyalgia

Myalgic Encephalomyelitis

Chronic Fatigue Syndrome

Medically Unexplained Physical Symptoms, MUPS

Long Covid and other post-viral syndromes.

Prolonged Convalescence

Multi Systemic Infectious Disease Syndrome, MSIDS

Debilitating Symptom Complexes attributed to Ticks - DSCATT

Chronic Lyme

This same syndrome may be caused by certain organic diseases, drugs and environmental toxins. (See Chapter 8)

A number of these patients who have not previously had Lyme disease or who have false positive tests are said to have "Chronic Lyme" disease. The furore over this is extreme.

In the diagnosis, treatment and understanding of the Lyme pandemic, Medicine with a capital 'M' conforms to the standards of Scientific proof that have guided it for the last one hundred years.

Thirty-two Professors of Medicine from Harvard, Yale, New York University, Duke, Johns Hopkins and across the United States; Neurologists, Pediatricians, Infectious Disease Specialists, Rheumatologists, Epidemiologists, got together to write the guidelines for the Prevention, Diagnosis and treatment of Lyme Disease. The last edition was published in 2020. For each of its sixty-four recommendations it summarizes the evidence, explains the rationale for the recommendation, and best of all, describes where the gaps in our knowledge are.

On the question of Chronic Lyme, they say this:

"*Chronic Lyme disease* lacks an accepted definition for either clinical use or scientific study."

"When evaluating such patients, clinicians should conduct a thorough and individualized history, physical evaluation, and appropriate laboratory investigations to identify whenever possible, the best fitting diagnosis."

"Prolonged antibiotic therapy is not helpful and may cause harm."

Now why would they write something like that when the Lyme 'Alternatives' have clinics full of people with Chronic Lyme Disease, who need treatment with intravenous antibiotics for six months to a year or longer? The only possible explanation is that these doctors, these *professors,* are in a conspiracy with the insurance companies and are obviously taking bribes from them to falsify their recommendations. Let's take them to court.

In Torrey vs. IDSA et al, twenty-eight patients sued six of the guidelines' authors and several insurance companies in 2017 for colluding to deny patients appropriate medical treatment. Within a month, the charges were dropped against the six authors, which included Allen Steere and continued against the IDSA as an organization.

The federal judge found that the plaintiffs had produced no evidence to support their conspiracy claims. The plaintiffs' accusations of fraud were similarly dismissed.

There exists a parallel universe. ILADS. It has its own society and its own guidelines and publishes research, sometimes scientific, sometimes not. It holds meetings, publishes journals and eerily resembles what in most countries would seem like the Medical Organization. Yet one already exists. It is generally accepted by politicians, the media and significant numbers of patients as being equivalent to or authentically in opposition to the establishment Medical Organization.

This is unique in the History of Medicine.

What's the difference between the two universes?

Some have argued that the entire rationale for ILADS existence is to allow profits to be made from long courses of antibiotics. Nutritional supplements are also supplied and un-approved blood tests are performed at a definite cost.

When the bill comes in, blame the Insurance companies for not covering the cost.

What it is *not* is a disagreement between two scientific viewpoints. For the scientific community, chronic lyme is ill defined, non specific and why is Lyme singled out?

The Exhaustion syndrome, what you call chronic lyme may follow practically any severe infection, some more than others. Look at Long Covid.

Here's the ILADS definition;

'For the purposes of the ILADS guidelines, "chronic Lyme disease "is inclusive of persistent symptomatologies including fatigue, cognitive dysfunction, headache, sleep disturbance and other neurologic features such as demyelinating disease, peripheral neuropathy and sometimes motor neuron disease, neuropsychiatric presentations, cardiac presentations (including electrical conduction delays and dilated cardiomyopathy) and musculoskeletal problems.'

This is too broad to be useful. *Borrelia burgdorferi* is not mentioned.

An analysis of USA (IDSA) guidelines together with French, Canadian, Swiss, Belgian, Swedish, Polish, German and United Kingdom medical association guidelines showed that none of them represented "chronic Lyme disease" as an entity and none of them recommend courses of antibiotics longer than one month.

This debate or debacle is such that it may take you over. Preoccupy you. "What's the matter with you doctors and your Lyme Wars?" as my next-door neighbor said to me as we were talking over the fence.

Let's get back to Lyme.

What must the practitioner do?

1. Have a high index of suspicion for acute, early disseminated and late disseminated Lyme. The earlier you make the diagnosis the better it is for the patient.

2. Although 75% of patients diagnosed with acute Lyme have EM, be aware that only one in ten are a bullseye and the typical rash is a filled in circle.

3. Absence of an EM rash, filled in or bullseye does not rule out Lyme

4. The antibody test is negative for the first two months of the infection.

5. Lyme may present as a flu like illness without a rash.

6. Since acute Lyme is more successfully treated than the late forms, and since neglected Lyme can have serious later consequences it makes sense to have a low threshold for treating patients with two to four weeks of doxycycline 100mgs twice daily. Why two to four? As a standard I give three weeks. The recommendation allows flexibility for the severity of the infection.

7. If the likelihood of Lyme is considered to be low, an alternate strategy is to wait two months and then perform an antibody test. This demands reliable cooperation from the patient

Later Forms

1. The presence of facial palsy or monoarthritis or symptoms and signs of meningitis, or typical skin rashes will be straightforward indicators of Lyme disease.

2. Less frequent complaints should alert the clinician. Cardiac complaints, particularly in younger patients, should make the practitioner immediately reach for his Lyme test kit. Dysrhythmias, particularly heart block, but also atrial fibrillation with a normal ventricular rate, palpitations and evidence of heart failure. This is amongst the most critical manifestation of Lyme to diagnose early as it is in heart disease that its mortality is predominantly found.

3. Look for Lyme in patients with unexplained conjunctivitis, uveitis, eye disease, chronic skin lesions, hearing loss, tinnitus, tiredness.

4. No diagnosis of dementia should be made without excluding Lyme disease by means of a spinal tap if necessary.

5. Particular care must be taken with neurological symptoms, which are common in early disseminated and late Lyme. Change in mental state, cognitive impairment, anxiety or depression, peripheral neuropathy and radiculopathy should arouse suspicion. All you have to do is order a test. And perhaps do a spinal tap.

An empathetic clinical attitude to patients with Lyme will go a long way towards making up for less than perfect tests and therapies.

What must the patient do?

1. Find a board-certified Infectious Disease doctor with whom you have a positive relationship.

2. Feel free to ask whatever questions come to mind in anticipation of a clear concise reply.

3. Try to avoid doctors that don't take insurance.

BIBLIOGRAPHY

Works can be broadly classified into three groups;

1. How I lived with Lyme and was misdiagnosed by the medical profession.

The Widening Circle. Polly Murray. 1996. Hardback. St Martin's Press. ISBN 978-0-312-14068-7

A patient, living in Lyme Connecticut, describes her determination to find out what is wrong with her. She makes little progress until Dr Allan Steere, becomes her physician. Who just happens to be the man who first described Lyme disease on the North American continent. In 1975 she was one of the first people to be diagnosed with the disease in the USA.

This book was published 26 years ago. It is historically significant, and an entertaining read, yet with increasing knowledge, much has changed, mostly for the better.

Lyme Disease. Amy Tan. 2004. An essay on her website.

http://www.amytan.net/lyme-disease.html

Amy Tan acquired Lyme disease and was misdiagnosed. Errors made by doctors drive patients into the arms of alternative practitioners. This should be required reading for medical students and doctors.

Cure Unknown: Inside the Lyme Epidemic. Pamela Weintraub. 2008. ISBN 978-0312378134

An outdated account of Lyme. However, she notices that the physicians with most experience were suburban or rural and therefore less influential than the professors at the medical centers who rarely saw the disease.

Believe Me. Yolanda Hadid. 2017. Hardback. St Martin's Press. ISBN 9781250132772

One of the "Real Housewives of Beverly Hills," Ms. Hadid has described what Lyme is like amongst the ultra-rich.

Sick: A Memoir. Porochista Khakpoor. 2018. Cannongate Books Ltd. ISBN 9781786896049

This book generalizes. Medicine is racist. Medicine discriminates against women. The medical profession would prefer to diagnose a psychiatric disease because it's cheaper than an organic one. Patients should take a lawyer with them on office visits with doctors.

The Lady's Handbook for her Mysterious Illness. Sarah Ramey. Doubleday. ISBN 978-0-7481-2591-3

This humorous-serious book points out that people call you names. Hypochondriac, malingerer, fibber, yuppie flu-er. Oh, for the name of a real disease! Myalgic encephalomyelitis! At last! She is 31 yrs. old and has suffered from a chronic illness for 17 years, that not only has no name it leaves no mark upon the body, and causes no detectable abnormality. Her insights are valuable to physicians. I can see her giving a course at medical school; mysterious Illnesses, four lectures.

2. Alternative treatments for Lyme.

The most important book in this group is by Richard Horowitz who may be considered the most influential alternative(-to-the-orthodox-medical-profession) physician.

Why Can't I Get Better? Richard Horowitz MD. 2013. Macmillan. USA. ISBN 9781250019400

Dr Horowitz describes himself as one of the country's foremost doctors.

He describes what is absolutely the correct approach to exhaustion. Augment the history with a detailed questionnaire, get to know the patient as well as you can and listen for as long as it takes. Exclude organic disease. His clinical approach is to look hard and meticulously for causes of the Exhaustion syndrome. If he cannot find a cause, or multiple causes, he then calls it Chronic Lyme.

Healing Lyme: Natural Healing of Lyme Borreliosis and the Coinfections Chlamydia and Spotted Fever Rickettsiosis, 2nd Edition. Stephen Harrod Buhner. 2015. Raven Press ISBN 9780970869647

Mr. Buhner has written an encyclopedic analysis of everything to do with Lyme Including a herbal assessment. *Astragalus propinquus* protects the immune system and overall, *Polygonum cuspidatum*, Japanese knotweed is the most useful herb for treating Lyme.

3. Statements of reality.

The Lyme Wars. Michael Specter. 2013. The New Yorker.

From this, the phrase Lyme Wars became widely used. He writes "I have an instinctive loathing for the middle ground, but that area, somewhere between the medical establishment and the activists is where I find myself."

Biography of a Germ. Arno Karlen 2001. Anchor books of Random House ISBN 0-385-72066-1

The germ in question is *Borrelia burgdorferi*. Interesting account of the organism in a conversational style.

The Infectious Disease Society of America. IDSA, AAN, and ACR Release Guidelines for Prevention, Diagnosis, and Treatment of Lyme Disease. 2020.

Written by thirty-four professors of medicine, Infectious Disease, Neurology, Rheumatology from A ranking medical schools.

Those who consider this document to be the work of the devil have not, I venture to suggest, read it.

It is a masterpiece of clarity and humility. I include this in the bibliography because it is surprisingly readable.

Recommendations are made with the evidence that supports them, which may be detailed as full or partial. The writers go out of their way to identify knowledge gaps and areas where there is need for further research. Like most guidelines, it also emphasizes that they are just that, and the physician in charge of the patient is the only one in a position to know when to accept and when to modify the recommendations.

Conquering Lyme Disease. Science bridges the great divide. Brian A Fallon MD and Jennifer Slotsky MD. 2019. *Columbia University Press. ISBN 9780231183857*

Authored by a scientist physician at Columbia Presbyterian Hospital in New York City, and a doctor in residency training with a degree in creative writing this is a detailed account of the issues and the evidence and is mandated reading. It is particularly good at analyzing the clinical trials that have been performed, including some of his own, and emphasizes yet again that Science is only way to bring the Lyme Wars to an end.

What Patients Say, What Doctors Hear by Danielle Offri MD.

A complete account of the doctor-patient relationship

REFERENCES

Afari Maxwell, E., F. Marmoush, M. U. Rehman, U. Gorsi, and F. J. Yammine. 2016. "Lyme Carditis: An Interesting Trip to Third-Degree Heart Block and Back." Case Reports in Cardiology. 5: 1–3.

Afzelius, A. 1921. "Erythema Chronicum Migrans." Acta Dermato-Venereol. 2: 120–25.

Arnold, L. M., J. I. Hudson, E. V. Hess, A. E. Ware, D. A. Fritz, M. B. Auchenbach, L. O. Starck, and P. E. Keck Jr. 2004. "Family Study of Fibromyalgia." Arthritis Rheum. 50, no. 3: 944–52.

Aucott, J. N., A. W. Rebman, L. A. Crowder, and K. B. Kortte. 2013. "Post-Treatment Lyme Disease Syndrome Symptomatology and the Impact on Life Functioning: Is There Something Here?" Quality of Life Research. 22: 75–84.

Auwaerter, P. G., J. S. Bakken, R. J. Dattwyler, J. S. Dumler, J. J. Halperin, E. McSweegan, R. B. Nadelman, S. O'Connell, E. D. Shapiro, S. K. Sood, A. C. Steere, A. Weinstein, and G. P. Wormser. 2011, September. "Antiscience and Ethical Concerns Associated with Advocacy of Lyme Disease." Lancet Infect Dis. 11, no. 9: 713–19.

Bannwarth, A. 1941. "Chronische Lymphocytäre Meningitis, Entzündliche Polyneuritis und Rheumatismus." Archive für psychiatrie und Nervenkrankheiten. 113: 284–376.

Barthold, S. 2012. "Persistence of Non-Cultivable Borrelia burgdorferi Following Antibiotic Treatment." In Global Challenges in Diagnosing and Managing Lyme Disease—Closing Knowledge Gaps: Hearing before the Subcommittee on Africa, Global Health, and Human Rights of the Committee on Foreign Affairs House of Representatives, 112 Cong., 2nd sess., July 17, Serial No. 112-169: 10–23.

Clark, K.L., Villegas Nunez, J.2023 "Detection of *Bartonella* DNA in Yellow Flies, Lone Star Ticks, and a Human Patient with Concurrent Evidence of Borrelia burgdorferi Infection in Northeast Florida, USA." Vector-Borne and Zoonotic Diseases, Vol. 23, No.8 **Published Online:** 1 Aug 2023 https://doi.org/10.1089/vbz.2023.0005

De Filippis, I., McKee, M.L. "Molecular typing in Bacterial Infections." Humana Press. ISBN 978-1627031844

Fallon, B. A., E. S. Levin, P. J. Schweitzer, and D. Hardesty. 2010, March. "The Underdiagnosis of Neuropsychiatric Lyme Disease in Children and Adults." Psychiatr Clin North Am. 21, no. 3: 693–703, viii.

Fallon, B. A., M. Pavlicova, S. W. Coffino, and C. Brenner. 2014. "Repeated Antibiotic Treatment in Chronic Lyme Disease." Journal of Spirochetal Diseases. 6, no. 4: 94–102.

Fallon, Brian A.; Sotsky, Jennifer. Conquering Lyme Disease (pp. 387-408). Columbia University Press. Kindle Edition. 2018

Claire M. Fraser, Sherwood Casjens, Wai Mun Huang, Granger G. Sutton, Rebecca Clayton, Raju Lathigra, Owen White, Karen A. Ketchum, Robert Dodson, Erin K. Hickey, Michelle Gwinn, Brian Dougherty, Jean-Francois Tomb, Robert D. Fleischmann, Delwood Richardson, Jeremy Peterson, Anthony R. Kerlavage, John Quackenbush, Steven Salzberg, Mark Hanson, Rene van Vugt, Nanette Palmer, Mark D. Adams, Jeannine Gocayne, J. Craig Venter "Genomic Sequence of a Lyme Disease Spirochaete, B. burgdorferi." Nature. 390: 580–86.

Garcia-Monco, J. C., B. F. Villar, J. C. Alen, and J. L. Benach. 1990. "Borrelia in the Central Nervous System: Experimental and Clinical Evidence for Early Invasion." J Infect Dis. 161: 1187–93.

Garin, C., and C. Bujaudoux. 1922. "Paralysie par les Tiques." Journal dé Medecine, Lyon. 7: 765–67.

Goldenberg, J. Z., S. S. Ma, J. D. Saxton, M. R. Martzen, P. O. Vandvik, K. Thorlund, G. H. Guyatt, and B. C. Johnston. 2013. "Chronic Inflammatory Demyelinating Polyradiculoneuropathy (CIDP): Current Perspectives." Medicine Update. 22: 580–85.

Gow, J. W., S. Hagan, P. Herzyk, C. Cannon, P. O. Behan, and A. Chaudhuri. 2009. "A Gene Signature for Post-Infectious Chronic Fatigue Syndrome." BMC Med Genomics. 2: 38.

Gugliotta, J. L., H. K. Goethert, V. P. Berardi, and S. R. Telford III. 2013. "Meningoencephalitis from Borrelia miyamotoi in an Immunocompromised Patient." N Engl J Med. 368, no. 3: 240–45.

Heller, J., G. Holzer, and K. Schimrigk. 1990. "Immunological Differentiation between Neuroborreliosis and Multiple Sclerosis." J Neurol. 237, no. 8, 465–70.

Hellerstrom, S. 1930. "Erythema Chronicum Migrans Afzelii." Acta Derm Venereol (Stockh.). 1: 315–21.

Hess, A., J. Buchmann, U. K. Zettl, S. Henschel, D. Schlaefke, G. Grau, and R. Benecke. 1999. "Borrelia burgdorferi Central Nervous System Infection Presenting as an Organic Schizophrenia-Like Disorder." Biol Psychiatry. 45, no. 6: 795.

Hodzic, E., S. Feng, K. Holden, K. J. Freet, and S. W. Barthold. 2008. "Persistence of B. burgdorferi following Antibiotic Treatment in Mice." Antimicrob Agents Chemother. 52, no. 5: 1728–36.

Horowitz, R.I, Fallon, J, Freeman, P.R.

Comparison of the Efficacy of Longer versus Shorter Pulsed High Dose Dapsone Combination Therapy in the Treatment of Chronic Lyme Disease/Post Treatment Lyme Disease Syndrome with Bartonellosis and Associated Coinfections

Microorganisms, 2023 - mdpi.com

Horowitz, H. W., M. E. Aguero-Rosenfeld, D. Holmgren, D. McKenna, I. Schwartz, M. E. Cox, and G. P. Wormser. 2013. "Lyme Disease and Human Granulocytic Anaplasmosis Coinfection: Impact of Case Definition on Coinfection Rates and Illness Severity." Clin Infect Dis. 56, no. 1: 93–99.

Horowitz, I.R. "Why Can't I Get Better? Solving the Mystery of Lyme and Chronic Disease" Macmillan Press. 2013

Hughes, R. A. C., P. Bouche, D. R. Cornblath, E. Evers, R. D. M. Hadden, A. Hahn, I. Illa, C. L. Koski, J. M. Leger, E. Nobile-Orazio, J. Pollard, C. Sommer, P. Van den Bergh, P. A. van Doom, and I. N. van Schaik. 2006. "European Federation of Neurological Societies/Peripheral Nerve Society Guideline on Management of Chronic Inflammatory Demyelinating Polyradiculoneuropathy: Report of a Joint Task Force of the European Federation of Neurological Societies and the Peripheral Nerve Society." European J Neurology. 13: 326–32.

Ismail, N., K. C. Bloch, and J. W. Mcbride. 2010. "Human Ehrlichiosis and Anaplasmosis." Clin Lab Med. 30, no. 1: 261–92.

Jacek, E., B. A. Fallon, A. Chandra, M. K. Crow, G. P. Wormser, and A. Alaedini. 2013. "Increased IFNα Activity and Differential Antibody Response in Patients with a History of Lyme Disease and Persistent Cognitive Deficits." J Neuroimmunol. 255, no. 1–2: 85–91.

Jarvis, W. T. "Rife Devices." The National Council Against Health Fraud. http://www.ncahf.org/articles/o-r/rife.html.

Joseph, J. T., K. Purtill, S. J. Wong, J. Munoz, A. Teal, S. Madison-Antenucci, H. W. Horowitz, M. E. Aguero-Rosenfeld, J. M. Moore, C. Abramowsky, and G. P. Wormser. 2012. "Vertical Transmission of Babesia microti, United States." Emerging Infect Dis. 18, no. 8: 1318–21.

Johnson, L., and R. B. Stricker. 2010, June. "The Infectious Diseases Society of America Lyme Guidelines: A Cautionary Tale about the Development of Clinical Practice Guidelines." Philos Ethics Humanit Med. 9, no. 5: 1–17. ——. 2004,

Jowett, N., R. A. Gaudin, C. A. Banks, and T. A. Hadlock. 2017. "Steroid Use in Lyme Disease-Associated Facial Palsy Is Associated with Worse Long-Term Outcomes." Laryngoscope. 127, no. 6: 1451–1458.

Kanjwal, K., B. Karabin, Y. Kanjwal, and B. P. Grubb. 2011. "Postural Orthostatic Tachycardia Syndrome following Lyme Disease." Cardiol J. 18, no. 1: 63–66.

Kaplan, R. F. and L. Jones-Woodward. 1997, March. "Lyme Encephalopathy: A Neuropsychological Perspective." Semin Neurol. 17, no. 1: 31–37.

Kilpatrick, H. J., A. M. LaBonte, and K. C. Stafford. 2014. "The Relationship between Deer Density, Tick Abundance, and Human Cases of Lyme Disease in a Residential Community." J Med Entomol. 51, no. 4: 777–84.

Klempner, M. S., L.T. Hu, J. Evans, C. H. Schmid, G. M. Johnson, R. P. Trevino, D. Norton, L. Levy, D. Wall, J. McCall, M. Kosinski, and Weinstein A. 2001a. "Two Controlled Trials of Antibiotic Treatment in Patients with Persistent Symptoms and a History of Lyme Disease." N Engl J Med. 345, no. 2: 85–92.

Klempner, M. S., P. J. Baker, E. D. Shapiro, A. Marques, R. J. Dattwyler, J. J. Halperin, and G. P. Wormser. 2013. "Treatment Trials for Post-Lyme Disease Symptoms Revisited." Am J Med. 126, no. 8: 665–69.

Klempner, M. S., R. Noring, and R. A. Rogers. 1993. "Invasion of Human Skin Fibroblasts by the Lyme Disease Spirochete, Borrelia burgdorferi." J Infect Dis. 167, no. 5: 1074–81.

Kowalski, T. J., S. Tata, W. Berth, M. A. Mathiason, and W. A. Agger. 2010. "Antibiotic Treatment Duration and Long-Term Outcomes of Patients with Early Lyme Disease from a Lyme Disease-Hyperendemic Area." Clin Infect Dis. 50, no. 4: 512–20.

Krause, P. J., S. Narasimhan, G. P. Wormser, L. Rollend, E. Fikrig, T. Lepore, A. Barbour, and D. Fish. 2013. "Human Borrelia miyamotoi Infection in the United States. N Engl J Med. 368, no. 3: 291–93.

Krause, P. J., D. Fish, S. Narasimhan, and A. G. Barbour. 2015. "Borrelia Miyamotoi Infection in Nature and in Humans." Clin Microbiol Infect. 21, no. 7: 631–39.

Krause, P. J., K. McKay, C. A. Thompson, V. K. Sikand, R. Lentz, T. Lepore, L. Closter, D. Christianson, S. R. Telford, D. Persing, J. D. Radolf, and A. Spielman; Deer-Associated Infection Study Group. 2002. "Disease-Specific Diagnosis of Coinfecting Tickborne Zoonoses: Babesiosis, Human Granulocytic Ehrlichiosis, and Lyme Disease." Clin Infect Dis. 34, no. 9: 1184–81.

Krupp, L. B., L. G. Hyman, R. Grimson, P. K. Coyle, P. Melville, S. Ahnn, R. Dattwyler, and B. Chandler. 2003. "Study and Treatment of Post Lyme Disease (STOP-LD): A Randomized Double Masked Clinical Trial." Neurology. 60, no. 12: 1923–30.

Kullberg, B. J., A. Berende, and A. W. Evers. 2016. "Longer-Term Therapy for Symptoms Attributed to Lyme Disease." N Engl J Med 375, no. 10: 998.

Lagunova, E.K., Liapunova, N.A. Tuul, D. Otgonsuren G. Co-infections with multiple pathogens in natural populations of *Ixodes persulcatus* ticks in Mongolia.

Parasites & vectors, 2022 – Springer

Lakos, A., and N. Solymosi. 2010. "Maternal Lyme Borreliosis and Pregnancy Outcome." Int J Infect Dis. 14, no. 6: e494–8.

Lantos, PM, Wormser, GP. Chronic co-infections in patients diagnosed with chronic Lyme disease: a systematic review. The American journal of medicine, 2014 - Elsevier

Larun, L., K. G. Brurberg, J. Odgaard-Jensen, and J. R. Price. 2016, February 7. "Exercise Therapy for Chronic Fatigue Syndrome." Cochrane Database Syst Rev. 2: CD003200. doi: 10.1002/14651858.CD003200.pub4.

Lawrence, C., R. B. Lipton, F. D. Lowy, and P. K. Coyle. 1995. "Seronegative Chronic Relapsing Neuroborreliosis." Eur Neurol. 35, no. 2: 113–17.

Lee, M., S. Silverman, H. Hansen, V. B. Patel, and L. Manchikanti. 2011. "A Comprehensive Review of Opioid-Induced Hyperalgesia." Pain Physician. 14: 145–61.

Li, X., G. A. McHugh, N. Damie, V. K. Sikand, L. Glickstein, and A. C. Steere. 2011. "Burden and Viability of Borrelia burgdorferi in Skin and Joints of Patients with Erythema Migrans or Lyme Arthritis." Arthritis Rheum. 63, no. 8: 2238–47.

Liegner, K. B., P. Duray, M. Agricola, C. Rosenkilde, L. A. Yannuzzi, M. Ziska, R. Tilton, D. Hulinska, J. Hubbard, and B. A. Fallon. 1997. "Lyme Disease and the Clinical Spectrum of Antibiotic Responsive Chronic Meningoencephalitis." J Spirochetal and Tick-Borne Diseases. 4: 61–73.

Lindquist, L. and O. Vapalahti. 2008. "Tick-Borne Encephalitis." Lancet. 371, no. 9627: 1861–71.

Livengood, J. A. and R. D. Gilmore, Jr. 2006. "Invasion of Human Neuronal and Glial Cells by an Infectious Strain of Borrelia burgdorferi." Microbes Infect. 8, nos. 14–15: 2832–840.

Logigian, E. L., R. F. Kaplan, and A. C. Steere. 1990. "Chronic Neurologic Manifestations of Lyme Disease." N Engl J Med. 323, no. 2:1438–44.

Logigian, E. L., R. F. Kaplan, and A. C. Steere. 1999. "Successful Treatment of Lyme Encephalopathy with Intravenous Ceftriaxone." J Infect Dis. 180: 377–83.

Macdonald, A. B. 1986. "Human Fetal Borreliosis, Toxemia of Pregnancy, and Fetal Death." Zentralbl Bakteriol Mikrobiol Hyg A. 263, nos. 1–2: 189–200.

Marchand, W. R. 2014. "Neural Mechanisms of Mindfulness and Meditation: Evidence from Neuroimaging Studies. World J Radiol. 6, no.7: 471–79.

Markowitz, L. E., A. C. Steere, J. L. Benach, J. D. Slade, and C. V. Broome. 1986. "Lyme Disease During Pregnancy." JAMA. 255, no. 24: 3394–96.

Marques, A. 2008. "Chronic Lyme Disease: An Appraisal." Infec Dis Clin North Am. 22: 341–60. Marques, A. R. 2015. "Laboratory Diagnosis of Lyme Disease – Advances and Challenges." Infect Dis Clin North Am. 29, no. 2: 295–307.

Marques, A., S. R. Telford III, S. P. Turk, E. Chung, C. Williams, K. Dardick, P. J. Krause, C. Brandeburg, C. D. Crowder, H. E. Carolan, M. W. Eshoo, P. A. Shaw, and L. T. Hu. 2014. "Xenodiagnosis to Detect B. burgdorferi Infection: A First-in-Human Study." Clin Infect Dis. 58, no. 7: 937–45.

Masters, E. J., C. N. Grigery, and R. W. Masters. 2008. "STARI, or Master's Disease: Lone Star Tick-Vectored Lyme-Like Illness." Infect Dis Clin North Am. 22, no. 2: 361–76.

Mathey, E. K., S. B. Park, R. A. C. Hughes, J. D. Pollard, P. J. Armati, M. H. Barnett, B. V. Taylor, P. J. B. Dyck, M. C. Kiernan, and C. S-Y Lin. 2015. "Chronic Inflammatory Demyelinating Polyradiculoneuropathy: From Pathology to Phenotype." J Neurol Neurosurg Psychiatry. 86: 973–85.

Mayberg, H. S., P. Riva-Posse, and A. L. Crowell. 2016, May 1. "Deep Brain Stimulation for Depression: Keeping an Eye on a Moving Target." JAMA Psychiatry. 73, no. 5: 439–40. Mayo Clinic. 2012, August 20. "Tularemia." Retrieved August 13, 2013. mayoclinic.com/health/tularemia/ds00714. McGuigan, M. A. 2012. "Chronic Poisoning: Trace Metals and Others." In Goldman's Cecil Medicine, 24th edition, edited by R. Cecil, L. Goldman, and A. Schafer. pp. 88–97. Philadelphia, PA: WB Saunders. Mead, P. 2004. Public Hearing on Lyme disease, State of Connecticut, Department of Public Health, January 29. http://www.ct.gov/ag/lib/ag/health/0129lyme.pdf.

Mead, P.S. 2015. "Epidemiology of Lyme Disease." Infect Dis Clin North Am. 29, no. 2: 187–210.

Meldrum, S. C., G. S. Birkhead, D. J. White, J. L. Benach, D, L. Morse. 1992. "Human Babesiosis in New York State: An Epidemiological Description of 136 Cases." Clin Infect Dis 15, no. 6: 1019-1023. https://doi.org/10.1093/clind/15.6.1019.

Murray, P. 1996. The Widening Circle: A Lyme Disease Pioneer Tells Her Story. New York: St. Martin's Press.

Mygland, A., U. Liøstad, V. Fingerle, T. Rupprecht, E. Schmutzhard, and I. Steiner; European Federation of Neurological Societies. 2010. "EFNS Guidelines on the Diagnosis and Management of European Lyme Neuroborreliosis." Eur J Neurol. 17, no. 1: 8–16.

Nadelman, R. B., J. Nowakowski, D. Fish, R. C. Falco, K. Freeman, D. McKenna, P. Welch, R. Marcus, M. E. Agüero-Rosenfeld, D. T. Dennis, and G. P. Wormser; Tick Bite Study Group. 2001. "Prophylaxis with Single-Dose Doxycycline for the Prevention of Lyme Disease After an Ixodes scapularis Tick Bite." N Engl J Med. 345, no. 2: 79–84.

Naro, A., D. Milardi, M. Russo, C. Terranova, V. Rizzo, A. Cacciola, S. Marino, R. S. Calabro, and A. Quartarone. 2016, July 27. "Non-Invasive Brain Stimulation, a Tool to Revert Maladaptive Plasticity in Neuropathic Pain." Front Hum Neurosci. https://doi.org/10.3389/fnhum.2016.00376.

Nelson, C., S. Elmendorf, and P. Mead. 2015. "Neoplasms Misdiagnosed as 'Chronic Lyme Disease.'" JAMA Intern Med. 175, no. 1: 132–33.

Nelson, C.A., S. Saha, K. J. Kugele, M. J. Delorey, M. B. Shankar, A. F. Hinckley, and P. S. Mead. 2015. "Incidence of Clinician-Diagnosed Lyme Disease, United States, 2005–2010." Emerg Infect Dis. 21, no. 9: 1625–31.

Nields, J. A., B. A. Fallon, and P. J. Jastreboff. 1999. "Carbamazepine in the Treatment of Lyme Disease-Induced Hyperacusis." J Neuropsychiatry Clin Neurosci. 11, no. 1: 97–99.

Nigrovic, L. E. and K. M. Thompson. 2007. "The Lyme Vaccine: A Cautionary Tale." Epidemiology and Infection. 135, no. 1: 1–8.

Norris, S. J. 2006. "Antigenic Variation with a Twist—the Borrelia Story." Mol Microbiol. 60, no. 6: 1319–22.

Oczko-Grzesik, B., and L. Kępa, Puszcz-Matlińska, M., Pudło, R., Żurek, A., & Badura-Głąbik, T. (2017). "Estimation of cognitive and affective disorders occurrence in patients with Lyme borreliosis. Ann Agric Environ Med. 24, no. 1: 33–38.

Oksi, J., M. Marjamaki, J. Nikoskelainen, and M. K. Viljanen. 1999. "B. burgdorferi Detected by Culture and PCR in Clinical Relapse of Disseminated Lyme Borreliosis." Ann Med. 31: 225–32.

Oksi, J., J. Nikoskelainen, H. Hiekkanen, A. Lauhio, M. Peltomaa, A. Pitkäranta, D. Nyman, H. Granlund, S. A. Carlsson, I. Seppälä, V. Valtonen, and M. Viljanen. 2007. "Duration of Antibiotic Treatment in Disseminated Lyme Borreliosis: A Double-Blind, Randomized, Placebo-Controlled, Multicenter Clinical Study." Eur J Clin Microbiol Infect Dis. 26, no. 8: 571–81.

Pachner, A. R. 1988. "Borrelia burgdorferi in the Nervous System: The New 'Great Imitator.'" Ann N Y Acad Sci. 539: 56–64.

Peeters, N., B. Y. van der Kolk, S. F. Thijsen, and D. R. Colnot. 2013. "Lyme Disease Associated with Sudden Sensorineural Hearing Loss: Case Report and Literature Review." Otol Neurotol. 34, no. 5: 832–37.

Plotkin, S. A. 2016. "Need for a New Lyme Disease Vaccine." N Engl J Med. 375, no. 10: 911–13.

Porcella, S. F. and T. G. Schwan. 2001. "Borrelia Burgdorferi and Treponema Pallidum: A Comparison of Functional Genomics, Environmental Adaptations, and Pathogenic Mechanisms." J Clin Invest. 107: 651–56.

Preac-Mursic, V., K. Weber, H. W. Pfister, B. Wilske, B. Gross, A. Baumann, and J. Prokop. 1989. "Survival of B. burgdorferi in Antibiotically Treated Patients with Lyme Borreliosis." Infection. 17: 355–59.

Pritt, B. S., P. S. Mead, D. K. Johnson, D. F. Neitzel, L.B. Respicio-Kingry, J. P. Davis, E. Schiffman, L. M. Sloan, M. E. Schriefer, A. J. Replogle, S. M. Paskewitz, J. A. Ray, J. Bjork, C. R. Steward, A. Deedon, X. Lee, L. C. Kingry, T. K. Miller, M. A. Feist, E. S. Theel, R. Patel, C. L. Irish, and J. M. Petersen. 2016. "Identification of a Novel Pathogenic Borrelia Species Causing Lyme Borreliosis with Unusually High Spirochaetaemia: A Descriptive Study." Lancet Infect Dis. 16: 556–64.

Rebman, A. W., J. N. Aucott, E. R. Weinstein, K. T. Bechtold, K. C. Smith, and L. Leonard. 2015. "Living in Limbo: Contested Narratives of Patients with Chronic Symptoms following Lyme Disease." Qual Health Research. 27, no. 4: 543–46.

Reis, C., M. Cote, D. Le Rhun, B. Lecuelle, M. L. Levin, M. Vayssier-Taussat, and S. I. Bonnet. 2011. "Vector Competence of the Tick Ixodes ricinus for Transmission of Bartonella birtlesii." PLoS Negl Trop Dis. 5, no. 5: e1186.

Romero, J. R., and K. A. Simonsen. 2008. "Powassan Encephalitis and Colorado Tick Fever." Infect Dis Clin North Am. 22, no. 3: 545–59.

Rothermel, H., T. R. Hedges, and A. C. Steere. 2001. "Optic Neuropathy in Children with Lyme Disease." Pediatrics. 108, no. 2: 477–81.

Rupprecht, T. A., M. Elstner, S. Weil, and H. W. Pfister. 2008. "Autoimmune-Mediated Polyneuropathy Triggered by Borrelial Infection?" Muscle Nerve. 37, no. 6: 781–85.

Sakkas, H., P. Gousia, V. Economou, V. Sakkas, S. Petsios, and C. Papadopoulou. 2016. "In Vitro Antimicrobial Activity of Five Essential Oils on Multidrug Resistant Gram-negative Clinical Isolates." J Intercult Ethnopharmacol. 5, no. 3: 212–18.

Sapi, E., S. L. Bastian, C. M. Mpoy, S. Scott, A. Rattelle, N. Pabbati, A. Poruri, D. Burugu, P. A. Theophilus, T. V. Pham, A. Datar, N. K. Dhaliwal, A. MacDonald, M. J. Rossi, S. K. Sinha, and D. F. Luecke. 2012. "Characterization of Biofilm Formation by B. burgdorferi in Vitro." PLoS ONE. 7, no. 10: e48277.

Schlesinger, P. A., P. H. Duray, P. A. Burke, A. C. Steere, and M. T. Stillman. 1985. "Maternal–Fetal Transmission of the Lyme Disease Spirochete, B. burgdorferi." Ann Intern Med. 103: 67–68.

Schutzer, S. E., T. E. Angel, T. Liu, A. A. Schepmoes, T. R. Clauss, J. N. Adkins, D. G. Camp, B. K. Holland, J. Bergquist, P. K. Coyle, R. D. Smith, B. A. Fallon, and B. H. Natelson. 2011. "Distinct Cerebrospinal Fluid Proteomes Differentiate Post-Treatment Lyme Disease from Chronic Fatigue Syndrome." PLoS ONE. 6, no. 2: e17287.

Skogman, B. H., K. Glimaker, M. Nordwall, M. Vrethem, L. Odkvist, & P. Forsberg. 2012. "Long-Term Clinical Outcome After Lyme Neuroborreliosis in Childhood." Pediatrics. 120, no. 2: 262–269.

Sharma, B., A. V. Brown, N. E. Matluck, L. T. Hu, and K. Lewis. 2015. "B. burgdorferi, the Causative Agent of Lyme Disease, Forms Drug-Tolerant Persister Cells." Antimicrob Agents Chemother. 59, no. 8: 4616–24.

Singh, S. K. and H. J. Girschick. 2004. "Molecular Survival Strategies of the Lyme Disease Spirochete B. burgdorferi." Lancet Infect Dis. 4, no. 9: 575–83.

Soloski, M. J., L. A. Crowder, L. J. Lahey, C. A. Wagner, W. H. Robinson, and J. N. Aucott. 2014. "Serum Inflammatory Mediators as Markers of Human Lyme Disease Activity." PLoS ONE. 9, no. 4: e93243.

Specter, M. 2013, July 1. "The Lyme Wars." The New Yorker.

Stanek G., J. Klein, R. Bittner, and D. Glogar. 1990. "Isolation of Borrelia Burgdorferi from the Myocardium of a Patient with Long-Standing Cardiomyopathy." N Engl J Med. 322, no. 4: 249–252.

Steere, A. C. and S. M. Angelis. 2006. "Therapy for Lyme Arthritis: Strategies for the Treatment of Antibiotic-Refractory Arthritis." Arthritis & Rheumatism. 54, no. 10: 3079–86.

Steere, A. C., P. H. Duray D. J. Kauffmann, and G.P. Wormser. 1985. "Unilateral Blindness Caused by Infection with the Lyme Disease Spirochete, Borrelia burgdorferi." Ann Inter Med. 103, no. 3: 382–84.

Steere, A. C., R. L. Grodzicki, A. N. Kornblatt, J. E. Craft, A. G. Barbour, W. Burgdorfer, G. P. Schmid, E. Johnson, and S. E. Malawista. 1983. "The Spirochetal Etiology of Lyme Disease." N Engl J Med. 308, no.13: 733–40.

Steere, A. C., S. E. Malawista, J. H. Newman, P. N. Spieler, and N. H. Bartenhagen. 1980, July. "Antibiotic Therapy in Lyme Disease." Ann Intern Med. 93, no. 1: 1–8.

Steere, A. C., R. T. Schoen, and E. Taylor. 1987. "The Clinical Evolution of Lyme Arthritis." Ann Intern Med. 107. no. 5: 725–31.

Steere, A. C. and V. K. Sikand. 2003. "The Presenting Manifestations of Lyme Disease and the Outcomes of Treatment." New Engl J Med. 348: 2472–74.

Steere, A. C., F. Strle, G. P. Wormser, L. T. Hu, J. A. Branda, J. W. R. Hovius, X. Li, and P. S. Mead. 2016. "Lyme Borreliosis." Nature Reviews: Disease Primers. 2: 1–18.

Strle, F., V. I. Maraspin, S. Lotric-Furian, E. Ruzić-Sabljić, and J. Cimperman. 1996. "Azithromycin and Doxycycline for Treatment of Borrelia Culture-Positive Erythema Migrans." Infection. 24: 64–68. Strle, F., V. Preac-Mursic, J. Cimperman, V. Ruzic E, Maraspin, M. Jereb. 1993. "Azithromycin versus Doxyxycline for Treatment of Erythema Migrans: Clinical and Microbiological Findings." Infection. 21, no. 2: 83–88.

Strle, F., E. Ruzić-Sabljić, J. Cimperman, S. Lotric-Furlan, and V. Maraspin. 2006. "Comparison of Findings for Patients with Borrelia garinii and Borrelia afzelii Isolated from Cerebrospinal Fluid." Clin Infect Dis. 43, no. 6: 704–10.

Strobino, B., S. Abid, and M. Gewitz 1999. "Maternal Lyme Disease and Congenital Heart Disease: A Case-Control Study in an Endemic Area." Am J Obstet Gynecol. 180: 711–16.

Strobino, B. A., C. L. Williams, S. Abid, R. Chalson, and P. Spierling. 1993. "Lyme Disease and Pregnancy Outcome: A Prospective Study of Two Thousand Prenatal Patients." Am J Obstet Gynecol. 169, no. 2, pt. 1: 367–74.

Telford, S. R., H. K. Goethert, P. J. Molloy, V. P. Berardi, H. R. Chowdri, J. L. Gugliotta, and T. J. Lepore. 2015. "Borrelia Miyamotoi Disease (BMD): Neither Lyme Disease Nor Relapsing Fever." Clin Lab Med. 35, no. 4: 867–82.

Tokarz, R., K. Jain, A. Bennett, T. Briese, and W. I. Lipkin. 2010. "Assessment of Polymicrobial Infections in Ticks in New York State." Vector Borne Zoonotic Dis. 10, no. 3: 217–21.

Topakian, R., K. Stieglbauer, K. Nussbaumer, and F. T. Aichner. 2008. "Cerebral Vasculitis and Stroke in Lyme Neuroborreliosis." Cerebrovascular Dis. 26: 455–61.

Tutolo, J. W., J. E. Staples, L. Sosa, and N. Bennett. 2017. "Notes from the Field: Powassan Virus Disease in an Infant—Connecticut, 2016." MMWR Morb Mortal Wkly Rep. 66, no. 15: 408–409. Uhde,

van Burgel, N. D., F. Bakels, A. C. Kroes, and A. P. van Dam. 2011. "Discriminating Lyme Neuroborreliosis from Other Neuroinflammatory Diseases by Levels of CXCL13 in Cerebrospinal Fluid." J Clin Microbiol. 49: 2027–30.

Vannier, E., B. E. Gewurz, and P. J. Krause. 2008. "Human Babesiosis." Infect Dis Clin North Am. 22, no. 3: 469–88. Vannier, E. and P. J. Krause. 2012. "Human Babesiosis." N Engl J Med. 366: 2397–407.

Wang, T. J., M. H. Liang, O. Sangha, C. B. Phillips, R. A. Lew, E. A. Wright, V. Berardi, A. H. Fossel, and N. A. Shadick. 2000. "Coexposure to Borrelia burgdorferi and Babesia microti Does Not Worsen the Long-Term Outcome of Lyme Disease." Clin Infect Dis. 31, no. 5: 1149–54.

Weintraub, P. 2013. "Cure Unknown: Inside the Lyme Epidemic". New York: St. Martin's Press.

Weissenbacher, S., J. Ring, and H. Hoffman. 2005. "Gabapentin for the Symptomatic Treatment of Chronic Neuropathic Pain in Patients with Late-Stage Lymeborreliosis: A Pilot Study." Dermatology. 211, no. 2: 123–27.

Williams, S. C., J. S. Ward, T. E. Worthley, and K. C. Stafford III. 2009, August. "Managing Japanese Barberry (Ranunculales: Berberidaceae) Infestations Reduces Blacklegged Tick (Acari: Ixodidae) Abundance and Infection Prevalence with B. burgdorferi (Spirochaetales: Spirochaetaceae)." Environ Entomol. 38, no. 4: 977–84.

Wormser, G. P., S. Bittker, D. Cooper, J. Nowakowski, R. B. Nadelman, and C. Pavia. 2001. "Yield of Large-Volume Blood Cultures in Patients with Early Lyme Disease." J Infect Dis. 184: 1070–72.

Wormser, G. P., E. Masters, D. Liveris, J. Nowakowski, R. B. Nadelman, D. Holmgren, S. Bittker, D. Cooper, G. Wang, and I. Schwartz. 2005. "Microbiologic Evaluation of Patients from Missouri with Erythema Migrans." Clin Infect Dis. 40, no. 3: 423–28. doi: 10.1086/427289.

Wormser, G. P., R. J. Dattwyler, E. D. Shapiro, J. J. Halperin, A. C. Steere, M. S. Klempner, P. J. Krause, J. S. Bakken, F. Strle, G. Stanek, L. Bockenstedt, D. Fish, J. S. Dumler, and R. B. Nadelman. 2006. "The Clinical Assessment, Treatment, and Prevention of Lyme Disease, Human Granulocytic Anaplasmosis, and Babesiosis: Clinical Practice Guidelines by the Infectious Diseases Society of America." Clin Infect Dis. 43, no. 9: 1089–134.

Wormser, G. P., Nadelman, R. J. Dattwyler, D. T. Dennis, E. D. Shapiro, A. C. Steere, T. J. Rush, D. W. Rahn, P. K. Coyle, D. H. Persing, D. Fish, and B. J. Luft. 2000. "Practice Guidelines for the Treatment of Lyme Disease." Clin Infect Dis. 31, Suppl 1: 1–14.

Printed in the United States
by Baker & Taylor Publisher Services